Contents

Key to symbols   v

1 Introduction   1
   1.1. Definition   1
   1.2. History and development   1

2 Production of antibodies   3
   2.1. Immunization   3
   2.2. Testing   4
   2.3. Region-specific antisera   4
   2.4. Monoclonal antibodies   5
   2.5. Characteristics of a 'good' antibody   6

3 Requirements for immunocytochemistry   8
   3.1. Insoluble and available antigen   8
   3.2. Visible end-product of reaction   12

4 Immunofluorescence methods   14
   4.1. Direct method   14
   4.2. Indirect method   14

5 Immunoenzyme methods   19
   5.1. Enzyme-conjugated antibody—indirect method   19
   5.2. The peroxidase anti-peroxidase method   20

6 Modifications of the basic methods   23
   6.1. Double or multiple staining   23
   6.2. Labelled-antigen methods   25
   6.3. Hapten-sandwich methods   25
   6.4. Gold-labelling methods   26
   6.5. Avidin—biotin methods   30

7 Specificity problems and essential controls   33
   7.1. Non-specificity of antisera   33
   7.2. Remedies for non-specificity due to heterogeneity of antibody   34
   7.3. Remedies for non-specificity due to cross-reactivity   35

Contents

8 *In vitro* methods for testing antibodies and checking antigens   37

   8.1. Enzyme-linked immunosorbent assay (ELISA)   37

   8.2. Radioimmunoassay   37

   8.3. Electroblot techniques   38

9 Applications of immunocytochemistry   39

   9.1. Histopathological diagnosis   39

   9.2. Quantification   40

   9.3. Basic research   41

   9.4. New imaging techniques   41

10 Microscopy   43

Appendix: technical notes   45

   A.1. Immunostaining by indirect method   45

   A.2. Peroxidase anti-peroxidase (PAP) method   46

   A.3. Cryostat sections   47

   A.4. Intensification of the peroxidase reaction   47

   A.5. Protease digestion   47

   A.6. To prevent sections becoming detached from slides   48

   A.7. Peroxidase development by alternatives to DAB methods   48

   A.8. Notes   49

   A.9. Development of alkaline phosphatase to give a blue end-product   49

   A.10. Post-embedding electron microscopical immunocytochemistry using an indirect immunogold method   50

References   52

Index   59

Figs. 7, 11 and 18 and Table 2 are adapted from Figs. 2.1, 2.2, 2.3, and Table 2.1 in Polak and Van Noorden (1983).

Key to symbols

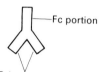

—Fc portion

Fab portions
(Two identical antigen-binding sites)

Immunoglobulin (antibody) molecule

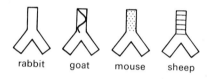

rabbit   goat   mouse   sheep

Species in which antibody is raised is indicated by the symbol in the Fc portion of the antibody

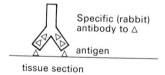

Specific (rabbit)
antibody to △

△ antigen

tissue section

Antigen specificity is indicated by the symbol in the Fab portion of the antibody and the substrate to which it binds.

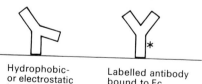

Hydrophobic-
or electrostatic
bonding of
immunoglobulin
to tissue

Labelled antibody
bound to Fc
receptors in tissue

Non-specific reactions

Key to symbols

Labels

$*$ Fluorophore (or other label)

$\bigcirc$ Peroxidase

$\bullet$ Insoluble end-product of peroxidase reaction (with H_2O_2 and DAB or other chromogen)

$\diamondsuit$ Alkaline phosphatase

$\blacklozenge$ End-product of alkaline phosphatase reaction (e.g. with naphthol phosphate and diazonium salt)

H   Hapten (as label)

     Colloidal gold particles

$\blacktriangledown$ Silver grains

Introduction

1.1. Definition

Immunocytochemistry is the use of labelled antibodies as specific reagents for the localization of tissue constituents (antigens) *in situ*.

1.2. History and development

The practice of immunocytochemistry originated with Albert H. Coons and his colleagues (Coons *et al.* 1941, 1955; Coons and Kaplan 1950) who were the first to label an antibody with a fluorescent dye, and use it to identify an antigen in tissue sections. As a result of this work, much of the uncertainty has now been removed from some aspects of histopathology, which were previously entirely dependent on special stains with interpretation sometimes precariously based on intuition and deduction. Because an antigen–antibody reaction is absolutely specific, positive identification of tissue constituents can now be achieved, although there are still problems, as will become apparent in the following pages.

The first fluorescent dye to be attached to an antibody was fluorescein isocyanate, but fluorescein isothiocyanate soon became the label of choice because the molecule was much easier to conjugate to the antibody. Fluorescein compounds emit a bright apple-green fluorescence when excited at a wavelength of 490 nm.

Following the early work and as better antibodies to more substances became available, the technique has been enormously expanded and developed. New labels have been introduced, for example, rhodamine isothiocyanate as an alternative, red, fluorescent dye and enzyme labels, visualized by established 'histochemical' techniques. The first enzyme to be used was peroxidase (Nakane and Pierce 1966; Avrameas and Uriel 1966). Other enzymes include alkaline phosphatase (Mason and Sammons 1978) and glucose oxidase (Suffin *et al.* 1979). The end-product of some of these enzyme reactions can be made electron-dense, but other, intrinsically electron-dense labels such as ferritin (Singer and Schick 1961) and colloidal gold (Faulk and Taylor 1971) have also been used to identify immunocytochemical reactions at the ultrastructural level. Antibodies have been labelled with radioactive elements, and the immunoreaction visualized by autoradiography, and some labels (e.g. latex particles) can even be used in scanning electron microscopy.

Among the techniques, the first modification of the original, directly-labelled antibody was the introduction of the indirect method (§ 4.2). This was followed by unlabelled antibody–enzyme methods which entirely avoided conjugation of a label to an antibody and the damage to its reactivity which that entailed. Other methods involved the use of a second antigen (hapten) as a label, visualized by a second antibody, the exploitation of the strong attraction between avidin and biotin, and numerous ways of improving the specificity and intensity of the final reaction and of carrying out multiple staining.

Some of these methods are described here, and the appendix gives practical details of the basic techniques. However, the subject is too vast to be covered completely in this handbook, which aims only to introduce the concept, and the reader is referred to several other useful publications which provide more detail on selected aspects (Sternberger 1979; Bullock and Petrusz 1982, 1983; Wick *et al.* 1982; Polak and Van Noorden 1983; 1986).

Production of antibodies

2.1. Immunization

Antibodies, which are mainly γ-globulins, are raised by immunizing rabbits (or guinea pigs, etc.) with antigen. The antigen must be completely pure or (preferably) synthetic to ensure as specific an antibody as possible. Despite this, the resulting antiserum will not be directed specifically and solely to the injected antigen. The antibodies produced will be directed to various parts of the antigen molecule and to the carrier protein, or parts of it. The donor animal serum will also contain many natural antibodies, which may react with tissue components. A positive-appearing immunoreaction cannot, therefore, be assumed to be due to the specific, desired antigen–antibody reaction unless stringent controls are carried out. It may be necessary to immunize many animals in order to end up with even one usable antiserum because little is known about what makes an animal react to a foreign protein and the production of antibodies is still a matter of chance.

If the antigen is large, for example an immunoglobulin, it can be used by itself to immunize an animal. If it is as small as many peptides or if the molecule is not itself immunogenic, it must be combined with a larger one for immunization. The small molecule (hapten) is chemically coupled (e.g. by glutaraldehyde or carbodiimide) to a larger 'carrier' protein molecule (e.g. limpet haemocyanin, thyroglobulin, or bovine serum albumin). The larger complex is a better stimulant of antibody formation than the small molecule alone. The donor animal's serum will contain a mixture of antibodies, reactive with different amino-acid sequences of the hapten and the carrier molecules, but the antibodies to the carrier molecule will either not react with the tissue to be stained (unless it were, for example, limpet tissue) or can be absorbed out, if necessary, by addition of the carrier protein, e.g. bovine albumin, to the antiserum prior to use. At an appropriate interval after the primary injection (subcutaneous), the rabbit (or guinea pig) is given a booster injection. Subsequently, blood is taken from it for testing for antibodies. No standard time course can be given for antibody raising, which is a highly individual procedure. The blood is then centrifuged to remove red blood cells. Although the antibody is contained in plasma which is not strictly serum since the fibrin has not been removed, the working solution is illogically known as an antiserum. For further reading on antibody production see Johnson and Thorpe, 1982

2.2. Testing

The next step is to test for the presence of antibody. The antiserum may be tested by the Enzyme-Linked ImmunoSorbent Assay (ELISA) against the pure antigen, or by radioimmunoassay (RIA) if there is one available or by a blotting technique (see p. 37 for these methods) but by far the most satisfactory way of testing for an antibody to be used in immunocytochemical staining is by immunocytochemistry on known positive tissue. This is because in the two *in vitro* methods mentioned above, pure antigen only is offered to the potential antiserum, and thus any interfering unwanted reactions due to the other constituents of the serum are not detected. By immunocytochemistry the antiserum may be evaluated for the quality of the specific staining against the 'background' and, if the background staining is unacceptably high and cannot be eliminated, the antiserum must be abandoned. Another reason for preferring an immunocytochemical test concerns the 'avidity' or 'stickiness' of the antibody (see p. 6). A useful antibody for immunocytochemistry must combine strongly with its antigen so as not to be washed off the tissue during the staining procedure.

In radioimmunoassay, competition takes place between radiolabelled and unlabelled antigen for binding to the antibody, leading to an equilibrium between the two, depending on the proportion of each available. However, a 'good' antibody for radioimmunoassay is often not 'good' for immunocytochemistry, and vice versa. The ELISA technique resembles the immunocytochemical technique more closely.

2.3. Region-specific antisera

The various couplers used react preferentially with different functional groups of the hapten molecule. Glutaraldehyde, for example, attaches primarily to amino groups. The free portion of the hapten molecule, distant from the combining site, is most likely to stimulate antibody formation; thus if the only free amino group in the hapten molecule is the $-NH_2$ terminal, then immunization with that hapten after coupling with glutaraldehyde is likely to produce antibodies to the 'free' C-terminal. Carbodiimide, on the other hand, will react with free amino or carboxyl groups; thus immunization with carbodiimide-coupled hapten, having these groups only at either end of the molecule, is likely to produce a mixture of antibodies directed to the C- and the N-terminals. A knowledge of the structure of the hapten is thus essential if the coupler is to be chosen intelligently so that the likely region-specificity of the resulting antibodies may be foreseen (Szelke 1983).

In the case of a peptide, it is often advantageous to have an antibody which is specific for only a certain area of the molecule; for instance, in cases where two peptides to be identified have amino-acid sequences in common and the antibody is required to distinguish between them (e.g. gastrin and cholecystokinin which share a C-terminal pentapeptide sequence). Most antibodies will only recognize sequences of four to eight amino acids. It is usually only by chance that a serum will contain antibodies to the desired part of the molecule. Attempts to characterize an antibody by assaying or absorbing against fragments of the antigen are not necessarily reliable because there is a danger that a small fragment of an antigen molecule in solution may lose the particular molecular configuration which gave it antigenicity when it was part of a whole molecule. Antigenic sites need not be straight-chain sequences of amino acids, but could be merely spatially adjacent sequences created by folding of the amino-acid chain. It is occasionally possible to use selected synthetic fragments of the molecule for immunization. With the proviso noted above, the resulting antiserum is then more likely to be specific for those fragments. Unfortunately, the smaller the amino-acid sequence used for immunization, the less immunogenic it is, so that the chances of obtaining a good antibody to a peptide fragment are slim. Another problem is that the shorter the amino-acid sequence, the more likely it is to be common to several different peptides. Thus, in peptide immunocytochemistry it is often essential to stain sections with antibodies to several different regions of the molecule, for example, to the N-terminal, mid-portion, and C-terminal amino acid sequences. Results of staining with such antibodies can confirm that the peptide being localized is the genuine molecule or suggest that a related, but not identical peptide is being identified (Larsson 1980).

2.4. Monoclonal antibodies

A method of obtaining 'pure' antibodies, even after immunization with a whole molecule, has recently been proposed by Milstein. (For a clear account of the development of the concept of monoclonal antibodies and their potential uses, see Milstein *et al.* 1979; Milstein 1980; McMichael and Fabre 1982.)

Antibodies are produced in mice, and lymphocytes from the spleen, source of the antibodies, are fused with mouse myeloma cells in culture. The fusion allows the hybrid cells to continue to grow and divide in culture and also to produce antibodies. One cell produces only one type of antibody and the cultured hybrid myeloma cells are gradually cloned into cell lines producing one antibody only. The procedure consists of screening the culture fluid from the various clones for antibody by radioimmunoassay, ELISA, or immunocytochemistry. For details of the production and testing of monoclonal antibodies see Ritter (1986). Antibodies specific to fragments of molecules could be produced in this way and, as the culture can be stored until further production is required, the method allows for a continuous supply of standard antibodies. The great advantage of monoclonal antibodies is their absolute specificity for a single sequence or 'epitope' on the antigen molecule. The problems associated with the multiple antibodies contained in polyclonal antisera thus do not arise and immunostained preparations are usually very clean. However, monospecificity for a particular epitope does not necessarily rule out cross-reactivity if the monoclonal antibody happens to be directed to an antigenic sequence shared by more than one substance, whether known or unsuspected, and in this case a monoclonal antibody would offer no advantage over a polyclonal one. A possible disadvantage of a monoclonal antibody derives from its very mono-specificity. A polyclonal antiserum is probably multivalent, consisting of anti-bodies to several regions of the antigen molecule, providing a strong detecting capacity. A monoclonal antibody, reactive with only one site on the molecule, may result in fewer antibody molecules being bound to the antigen and subsequently detected by the labelling method, resulting in weaker staining. Similarly, the one particular epitope of interest on the antigen molecule may be altered by fixation or processing so as to be unavailable for reaction so that no staining will be seen. This is why some monoclonal antibodies will only react with fresh or frozen material and not with fixed paraffin sections. A polyclonal antibody would have more chances of attaching to different epitopes on the molecule that might be less altered. One answer to this problem might be to use a 'cocktail' of monoclonal antibodies to different regions of the antigen molecule. Another possibility is to immunise with 'fixed' antigen. In any case, it is essential to screen antibodies in the system in which they are to be used (see § 2.2).

In addition to the use of monoclonal antibodies as pure antibodies to known antigens, monoclonal antibodies may be raised to unknown antigens and used as markers for particular cell types or cytoplasmic constituents. By immunizing mice with human thymocytes and cloning the antibodies produced, several series of monoclonal antibodies to human T lymphocytes have been produced which can be used to separate the cell types immunocytochemically (Kung *et al.* 1979). The antibodies act against constituents of membranes of the cells (Fig. 1).

Similarly, monoclonal antibodies separated from the antibodies resulting from immunization of mice with rat-brain homogenates are being used to study the relationships between different classes of brain cell (Sterberger 1983).

'Good' antibody characteristics (see § 2.5) apply to monoclonal as much as to polyclonal antibodies, but the availability of such highly specific tools has truly revolutionized immunocytochemistry and its applications in histopathology and cell biology (Gatter *et al.* 1985).

2.5. Characteristics of a 'good' antibody

The main requirement for a good antibody is that it shall be of high affinity for its antigen, in other words that its binding sites fit well with the antigenic sites on its specific antigen and do not attach to other antigens. The avidity, or binding strength, is a connected property depending on the number of fitting sites between the antigen and antibody (Roitt 1980). Immunocytochemistry requires antibodies of high avidity (stickiness) so that they are not washed off the section during the staining process.

It is useful to find that the unwanted antibodies in an antiserum are less avid than the antibody to the specific antigen and are, therefore, fortunately washed off the section during the staining procedure. However, it should be emphasized that great care must be taken when dealing with histological sections of abnormal or damaged tissue such as come to a routine histopathology department and with

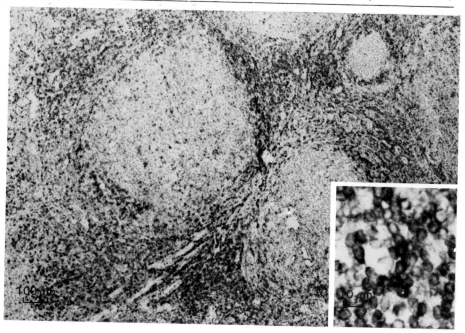

Fig. 1. Human tonsil immunostained by the indirect immunoperoxidase method using a mono-clonal antibody to T-lymphocyte cell membranes and a peroxidase-conjugated rabbit anti-mouse IgG. Preparation counterstained with haematoxylin. Note the distribution of the T cells in the paracortex with a few cells only in the follicle centre. The membrane localization is demonstrated in the inset. Tissue preparation: Cryostat section (4 μm) thoroughly air-dried, fixed for 10 minutes in 100 per cent ethanol at 4°C, and then transferred to phosphate-buffered saline without further drying.

whole cells in smears, because these preparations seem to attract and hold non-specific antibodies. Very thorough controls are essential for these, as for all, prep-arations.

The titre or concentration of the antibody is also very important. A high titre allows a high dilution which, in immunocytochemistry, means that the population of unwanted antibodies which might react with tissue components is diluted out. In radioimmunoassay, where the dilutions used are generally about 10 000 times higher than for immunocytochemistry, specific antigen only is offered to the antibody, so that unwanted reactions are ruled out. Nevertheless, a high dilution allows for removal of contaminating proteins and great economy in the use of labelled antigen which helps to eliminate 'noise' due to excess radioactivity. High dilutions are also advantageous in that they allow for the fullest use of the available quantity of good antibodies, which are expensive to produce. Unfortunately, the factors leading to antibodies of high avidity and titre are unknown.

If monoclonal antibodies are being used, the dilution factor becomes less import-ant as unwanted reactions are absent and there is theoretically an unlimited supply of antibody.

3

Requirements for immunocytochemistry

The essential conditions for immunocytochemistry are summarized in Table 1.

Table 1. *Essential conditions for immunocytochemistry*

1. Preservation of antigen (see Table 2, p. 9)
2. Specific staining (see Table 4, p. 36)
3. Well characterized antibody
4. Easily visible label

3.1. Insoluble and available antigen

Successful immunostaining requires tissue antigens to be made insoluble and yet their antigenic sites must be available to the applied antibody without great alteration of their tertiary structure. In addition, the tissue architecture must be preserved (fixed) so that the immunoreactive cell or organelle may be identified in context. It used to be thought that good tissue fixation meant poor antigen availability, due to the strong cross-linking of tissue proteins by the conventional aldehyde fixatives, but recent work indicates that such fixatives can be used, even, in some cases, with osmium tetroxide post-fixation for electron microscopy, provided that the correct pre-treatment is used. This advance is probably the result of generally improved antibodies and more rigorously controlled technique. Good preservation for most of the peptide hormones and neuropeptides can be achieved, without the need for further treatment, by freeze-drying the tissue and exposing it to the vapour of weakly cross-linking reagents such as formaldehyde, p-benzoquinone, or diethylpyrocarbonate (Pearse and Polak 1975) but this method does not provide good morphological preservation for electron microscopy. The embedding process, with impregnation of the tissue in hot wax or epoxy resin, may also damage the antigenicity of some peptides. Cryostat sections of frozen tissue, pre-fixed by immersion or perfusion in buffered formaldehyde or p-benzoquinone, are, therefore, preferred by some authors for light microscopical investigations, paticularly for peptide-containing nerves (Elde *et al.* 1976; Bishop *et al.* 1978). Methods of fixation and their uses are summarized in Table 2.

A recent report suggests that fixation of peptides with p-benzoquinone solution may be improved by using the fixative at a higher pH and temperature, e.g. pH 8.0 and 37°C, to improve its cross-linking reactivity, (Bu'Lock *et al.* 1982).

Fixation with formaldehyde may also be improved by altering the pH of the

Table 2. *Fixation*

Tissue preparation	Use
Smears or impressions of fresh tissue or cryostat sections of fresh-frozen tissue, unfixed or post-fixed in acetone, alcohol, etc.	Identification of autoimmune sera, cell surface antigens, extracellular antigens (e.g. immune deposits in glomerular basement membrane), tumour markers in cytological preparations
Cryostat sections or whole-mount preparations of tissue pre-fixed in para-benzoquinone or paraformaldehyde	Particularly useful for tracing antigens in nerves (e.g. peptides and amines)
Freeze-dried tissue, fixed in formal-dehyde or parabenzoquinone vapour and embedded in paraffin	Intracellular water-soluble antigens (e.g. peptides in endocrine cells)
Routine formaldehyde-containing fixatives; paraffin sections (preferably dried at 37°C). 'Over-fixed' antigenic sites may be revealed by pre-treatment of the sections with a proteolytic enzyme	Histopathological diagnosis (tumour markers, intracellular immunoglobulins, peptide hormones, etc.)
Periodate–lysine–paraformaldehyde; glutaraldehyde-based fixatives; resin-embedded, frozen, or vibratome sections.	Electron microscopical immunocytochemistry and light microscopical immunocyctochemistry on semi-thin sections.

solution. In the method reported by Berod *et al.* (1981) for localization of a diffusible antigen, tyrosine hydroxylase, formaldehyde was perfused at pH 6.5 for rapid penetration, although it fixes poorly at this pH. When the fixative was widely distributed, its pH was abruptly raised to 11 to increase the cross-linking reaction.

Pre-fixed cryostat sections, organ- or cell-culture preparations, smears, or whole-mount preparations which, unlike paraffin sections, have not been subjected to solvents during processing, often need to have the lipid components of the cell membranes broken down to improve penetration of the antibodies. This break-down may be achieved by soaking the preparations in a buffer containing a detergent such as Triton X-100 (0.2 per cent) or saponin before immunostaining. Larsson (1981) recommends this procedure for paraffin and resin sections as well, but in our experience, this is not necessary; however, addition of detergent to the rinsing buffer may help to prevent non-specific attachment of protein to the section.

An alternative method is to subject the preparations to dehydration through graded alcohols to xylene and then to rehydrate them before staining. The disadvantage of this method is that solvent-labile antigens may be leached out.

If the tissue to be processed contains a large amount of proteolytic enzymes (e.g. gut or pancreas), it may be found useful to include a proteinase-inhibitor such as trasylol in the fixative solution and the buffer rinse. The morphology of the tissue will probably be better and some labile peptides such as vasoactive intestinal polypeptide will stand a better chance of preservation.

Diethylpyrocarbonate and p-benzoquinone have not yet been tried to any extent as fixatives for cell surface or extracellular antigens, for which fresh-frozen cryostat sections are usually used, or for intracellular immunoglobulins, which can generally be shown in formalin-fixed material.

For electron microscopy, pre-embedding and post-embedding methods are available. Vibratome or cryostat sections of pre-fixed material may be immunostained, the reaction product being made electron-dense before the material is embedded in resin fo: the electron microscope. This method has the advantage that antigens are not exposed to solvents before immunostaining and that the immunostained area may be selected by light microscopy before embedding, but the disadvantage that adjacent thin sections cannot easily be stained by different antibodies. As mentioned above, some method of lipid breakdown should be incorporated when immunostaining these sections, but it need not be used for post-embedding staining of ultra-thin sections, in which the cell contents are exposed to the antibody.

The latest technology for electron microscopical immunocytochemistry provides for the preparation of ultra-thin sections of frozen, pre-fixed tissue (Tokuyasu 1980, 1983). These sections may be immunostained on grids without processing through solvents or resins and are particularly useful for fine structural localization of labile antigens.

Other fixatives have included a periodate/lysine/paraformaldehyde mixture (McLean and Nakane 1974) particularly for glycoproteins and a carbodiimide/glutaraldehyde mixture (Willingham 1980) for fibroblast constituents localized by ferritin. Fresh-frozen cryostat sections fixed in alcohol or acetone are useful for surface immunoglobulin antigens of lymphocytes (see Fig. 1). These methods have not been extensively used for peptides.

The method of choice depends on the antigen–antibody reaction to be carried out and the expected localization of the antigen. It is of great importance that the tissue be processed as freshly as possible, whether fixation is by immersion in solution or by vapour fixation after freeze-drying. In the latter case, once the tissue has been frozen, it may be stored at $-70°C$ for an indefinite period before drying.

Protease treatment

A little understood, but practical way of revealing strongly cross-linked peptides in conventionally formalin-fixed and paraffin-embedded material is to treat the sections with a protease such as trypsin or pronase (Huang *et al.* 1976) before immunostaining. It is thought that the protease treatment breaks the cross-linking bonds of the fixative with the protein to reveal the antigenic sites. Some antigens may be destroyed by the enzyme incubation and there is also a possibility that large protein molecules (e.g. precursors of bioactive peptides) may be cleaved to smaller molecules by the enzyme. If these molecules display antigenic sites that were not available on the precursor, a false positive stain may be achieved. However,

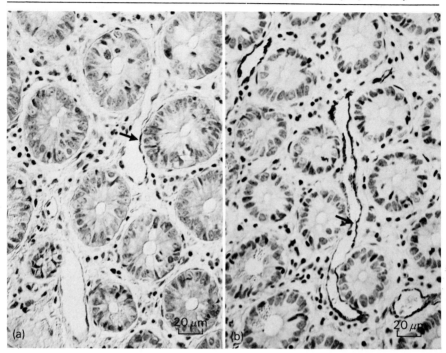

Fig. 2. Human duodenum immunostained for Factor VIII-related protein, a marker for endothelial cells, by the peroxidase anti-peroxidase method using a rabbit antibody to Factor VIII
followed by unconjugated goat anti-rabbit IgG, then rabbit PAP complex. The section shown in
(a) was stained without trypsin pretreatment, the adjacent section in (b) was stained after
'digestion' for 30 minutes at 37°C in 0.1 per cent trypsin in 0.1 per cent calcium chloride at
pH 7.8. Note the very slight reaction in the endothelial cells of the vessel wall in (a) compared
with the intense reaction in (b) (arrows). Counterstained with haematoxylin. Tissue preparation:
tissue fixed in neutral phosphate-buffered formalin and embedded in paraffin; 4 μm section.
Photographed with Nomarski interference-contrast optics.

bearing in mind these possibilities, protease pre-treatment should be tried routinely
whenever preliminary immunostaining is found to be inadequate (Fig. 2). A useful
discussion is that of Finley and Petrusz (1982). For practical details see § A5.

Oxidation treatment

Even conventional glutaraldehyde or paraformaldehyde–glutaraldehyde mixtures
have now been successfully used for a combination of immunocytochemistry and
electron microscopy. Ultra-thin sections of glutaraldehyde/osmium-fixed material
may also be used after oxidation with hydrogen peroxide (Baskin *et al.* 1979;
Beauvillain and Tramu 1980) or sodium metaperiodate (Bendayan and Zollinger
1982, 198).

Adherence of sections to slides

Paraffin sections for immunostaining should never be 'baked' on a hot plate as this destroys the antigenicity of many substances. They should be thoroughly dried (at least overnight) at $37°$C. In some cases no adhesive is necessary on the glass slide, but if protease digestion is to be used, or a particularly long method involving several steps and rinses, and essentially for pre-fixed cryostat sections, some form of adhesive is required. Albumen may be used for ordinary paraffin sections and cryostat sections may be mounted on formol–gelatine- or chrome–gelatine-treated slides but a better and universally applicable coating is provided by poly-L-lysine (Husain *et al.* 1980). High molecular-weight polymers of L-lysine (150 000–300 000) are the most effective (Huang *et al.* 1983). See § A.6 for method.

3.2. Visible end-product of reaction

The first labels were fluorescent and both fluorescein and tetramethyl rhodamine isothiocyanate have remained popular, giving intense green or red fluorescence, easily visible against a non-fluorescent background. A fluorescent counterstain may sometimes be useful to allow non-immunoreactive parts of the tissue to be seen. Evans blue and sometimes the periodic acid–Schiff method (Colour Plate 1, inside back cover) provide a red background to fluorescein fluorescence (though they may reduce the brightness of the specific fluorescence) and methyl green fluoresces red which can be useful as a nuclear counterstain.

Peroxidase or alkaline phosphatase-labelled antibodies have the advantage that an ordinary transmitted-light microscope can be used and the preparations are permanent. The development of the enzyme reaction is progressive and can be monitored and stopped when the 'signal-to-noise' ratio is adequate. The proportion of fluorescent or enzyme label to antibody used in conjugation must be carefully calculated. Antibody activity may be altered by an excess of label and unbound label must in any case be removed by dialysis or column chromatography before the antibody can be used. All the antibody molecules should be labelled as any unlabelled antibody present will compete for binding sites with the labelled antibody and reduce the visibility of the final reaction.

In addition to the unlabelled antibody–enzyme methods (§ 5.2) numerous ways of improving the visibility of the peroxidase reaction end-product have been suggested (see § A.4). In general, these enhancement methods improve the sensitivity of the reaction by allowing a smaller quantity of antigen in the tissue to be detected by the same concentration of antibody, or the specificity is improved by allowing the same quantity of antigen to be detected by a lower concentration of antibody, so that unwanted antibodies can be diluted further out of the incubation antiserum. Nuclear or other counterstains should be chosen to provide contrast to but not to detract from the impact of the immunostained product.

Immunogold staining (see p. 26) can be enhanced for the light microscope by using epipolarization microscopy (see Chapter 10) or by a new method of silver precipitation (Holgate *et al.* 1983*a*, *b*; Springall *et al.* 1984; Hacker *et al.* 1985). As regards electron microscopical immunocytochemistry, it is in part the greater contrast of the gold particles with conventionally counterstained preparations that gives colloidal gold its advantages as a label over osmicated DAB-developed peroxidase.

Labelling an antibody with fluorescein isothiocyanate (FITC) is done quite simply (see Sternberger 1979, for details). Briefly, the method consists of:

1. Isolation of IgG.
2. Reaction of the lgG with FITC in the right proportions at alkaline pH.
3. Separation of antibody from unconjugated FITC on a Sephadex G25 column.
4. Separation of labelled from unlabelled IgG on a DEAE cellulose column.

Labelling with peroxidase requires an additional large molecule such as glutaraldehyde to cross-link the enzyme to the antibody. The preparation of PAP is more complicated, as it involves purification of the complex. For labelling with gold, antibodies are attached to gold particles by non-covalent adsorption. A radioactive label may be incorporated within an antibody during its production, and thus the use of a conjugated label may be avoided. The site of reaction is identified by autoradiography (Cuello *et al.* 1982). Tritiated biotin (see § 6.5) provides another method of using autoradiography to identify immunoreactions (Hunt *et al.* 1986).

An easier way of obtaining these reagents is to buy them. Excellent fluorescent label- or enzyme-conjugated antibodies and enzyme anti-enzyme complexes can now be bought from many suppliers and gold-labelled reagents are also available. Although they are expensive, they are probably less so than the time and effort of preparing what might be inferior products.

All antibodies, whether home-made or commercially obtained, must be titrated before use in a known positive immunocytochemical system to find the best working dilution. This will also depend on the staining time. Short staining times (10 mins to 1 hour) require higher antibody concentrations than long (12–24 hours) and often result in more non-specific staining because the contaminating antibody sub-populations have not been diluted out.

4

Immunofluorescence methods

4.1. Direct method

In his original method Coons (Coons and Kaplan 1950) used a one-step (direct) staining method in which the specific antibody was conjugated to fluorescein isothiocyanate (FITC). The conjugated antiserum, diluted in phosphate-buffered saline (PBS), was allowed to react with a tissue section and the unbound antibody was then washed off with PBS. The section was examined in an ultraviolet microscope and the site of attachment of the antibody fluoresced apple green (Fig. 3).

4.2. Indirect method

The method was subsequently adapted to become the indirect immunofluorescence technique (Coons *et al.* 1955) which is still widely used (Figs. 4 and 5 and Colour Plate 1). In this method the primary antibody is not conjugated, but a second layer is added which consists of an antibody raised to the γ-globulin of the species which donated the first antibody, for example, goat anti-rabbit γ-globulin, which is conjugated with FITC. The first antibody, rabbit anti-antigen, which is bound to antigenic sites in the tissue section, then acts as a γ-globulin antigen for the second, fluorescent antibody (Fig. 6).

Advantages

1. Anti-IgG sera are usually hyperimmune and of very high avidity.
2. Two labelled anti-immunoglobulin molecules can bind to each primary antibody molecule, increasing the sensitivity of the reaction. For simplicity, only one is illustrated.
3. Economy. One fluorescent second-layer antibody can be used to stain any number of first-layer antibodies to different antigens, provided they have all been raised in the same species donating the IgG for the second-layer antibody. Conjugated second-layer antibodies are now widely available commercially. Other fluorescent labels such as rhodamine and Texas red which give a red fluorescence have also been used, but give less intense fluorescence than FITC. They are useful in double immunofluorescence techniques, and Texas red fades less rapidly than rhodamine.

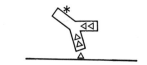

Specific antigen–antibody reaction
with labelled primary antibody

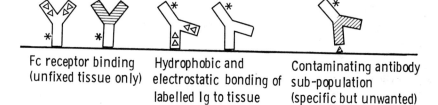

Fc receptor binding   Hydrophobic and   Contaminating antibody
(unfixed tissue only)   electrostatic bonding of   sub-population
                         labelled Ig to tissue   (specific but unwanted)

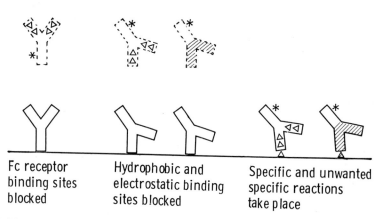

Fc receptor   Hydrophobic and   Specific and unwanted
binding sites   electrostatic binding   specific reactions
blocked   sites blocked   take place

Fig. 3. Direct method. Primary antibody conjugated with fluorescein (or peroxidase). Unwanted antibodies to tissue antigens and sub-populations of contaminating antibodies are also labelled. Some non-specific reactions due to these and to hydrophobic and electrostatic bonding of immunoglobulins to the tissue are also shown in (b), but may be partly prevented by incubating the section with unconjugated nonimmune serum from the antibody-donor species or with an inert protein such as albumin before incubation with the antibody (c). This method is useful for double staining with two primary antibodies separately labelled, for example, with rhodamine isothiocyanate and fluorescein isothiocynate (Valnes and Brandtzaeg 1982).

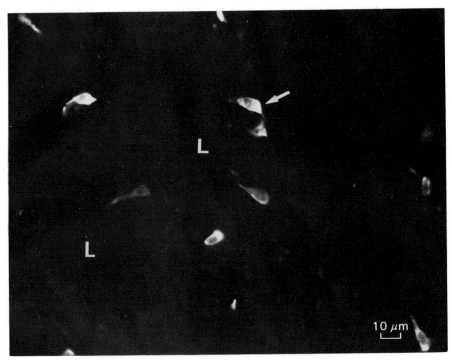

Fig. 4. Human colon immunostained by the indirect immunofluorescence method using rabbit anti-glucagon and fluorescein-conjugated goat anti-rabbit IgG to show the enteroglucagon cells. Note the base of the immunofluorescent cells resting on the basement membrane (arrow) and the apical processes extending towards the lumen (L). Tissue preparation. Tissue fixed in p-benzoquinone solution; cryostat section (6 μm).

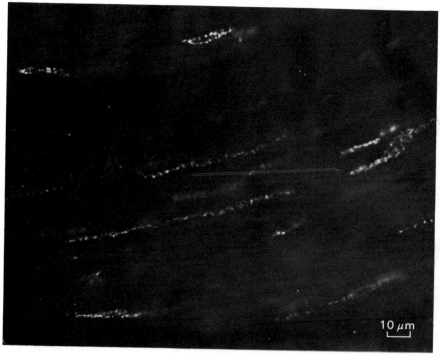

Fig. 5. Rat stomach immunostained by the indirect immunofluorescence method using rabbit anti-vasoactive intestinal polypeptide (VIP) and fluorescein-conjugated goat anti-rabbit IgG to show VIP-containing nerve fibres in the muscle of the stomach wall. Note the typical varicosities. VIP is a peptide neurotransmitter that promotes secretion, vasodilatation and muscle relaxation. Tissue preparation. Tissue fixed in p-benzoquinone solution; cryostat section (10 μm).

(a)

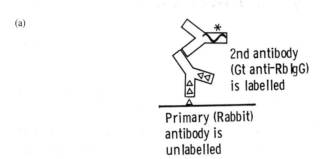

2nd antibody
(Gt anti-Rb IgG)
is labelled

Primary (Rabbit)
antibody is
unlabelled

(b)

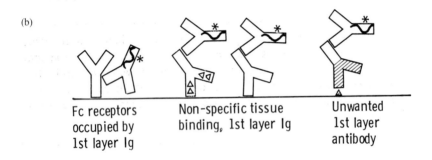

Fc receptors
occupied by
1st layer Ig

Non-specific tissue
binding, 1st layer Ig

Unwanted
1st layer
antibody

(c)

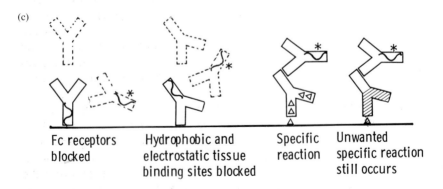

Fc receptors
blocked

Hydrophobic and
electrostatic tissue
binding sites blocked

Specific
reaction

Unwanted
specific reaction
still occurs

Fig. 6. Indirect method. Some non-specific tissue reactions which are included in (b) may
be prevented (c) by blocking with inert protein or with unconjugated non-immune serum
from the donor of the second-layer antibody prior to incubation with the primary antibody.

Immunoenzyme methods

5.1. Enzyme-conjugated antibody — indirect method

Peroxidase, first introduced by Nakane and Pierce (1966), has lately replaced fluorescein as the antibody label in many immunocytochemical reactions. The indirect method is carried out as indicated, but the antibody is visualized by a histochemical reaction for peroxidase, usually Graham and Karnovsky's (1966) diaminobenzidine (DAB) reaction.

Advantages

Permanent sections can be prepared which do not fade like the fluorescent sections, are visible with an ordinary microscope, and are much quicker to photograph. Stain deposits on fine nerve fibres are particularly easily seen with Nomarski interference optics. The peroxidase method can also be adapted for use at the ultrastructural level by treating the reaction product with osmium tetroxide which makes it electron-dense.

Disadvantages

The two extra stages with the extra washing steps, which are necessary in the technique, may result in the tissue becoming detached from the slide more often than in the fluorescent method and also make the method longer to carry out. The first of the extra steps is immersion of the section in a solution of hydrogen peroxide in buffer or methanol to 'exhaust' the endogenous peroxidase of the tissue, which might confuse the picture. As alternatives to hydrogen peroxide, the reaction may be blocked with periodate and borohydride (Heyderman 1979), sodium nitroferricyanide, or phenyl hydrazine (Straus 1971, 1972). The other extra step is the histochemical reaction of the peroxidase on the antibody. There is also evidence that prolonged exposure to benzidine, of which diaminobenzidine is a derivative, can be carcinogenic in man (International Agency for Research on Cancer 1972). It should be noted that the evidence comes from subjects suffering prolonged exposure to the compound during the industrial manufacturing process when concentrations are likely to be at far higher levels than would be derived from the 25 to 50 mg per cent solutions used in histochemistry. However, the experiments of Weisburger *et al.* (1978) indicated that the addition to benzidine of the two amino groups to form diaminobenzidine almost eliminated the carcinogenic effect

relative to benzidine. Nevertheless, precautions to prevent undue exposure and con-
tamination are advisable, e.g. keeping one area of the laboratory, preferably in a
fume cupboard, for the DAB development, wearing gloves when handling solutions
of DAB, and treating the solution with sodium hypochlorite (ordinary household
bleach) after it is finished with as well as glassware, instruments, and spills. DAB
solutions are most safely stored frozen in aliquots (see § A8). There are some
alternative reagents which are supposed to be less carcinogenic than DAB,
e.g. Hanker–Yates reagent, p-phenylene diamine with pyrocatechol (Hanker *et al.*
1977), or 3-amino-9-ethyl carbazole (Graham *et al.* 1965). However, a recent
note suggests that the latter substance may be carcinogenic and it is wise to take
precautions (Tubbs and Sheibani 1982). DAB is still the most widely used capture
reagent because it is extremely sensitive and the end-product is easy to see and
insoluble so that stained sections may be dehydrated and mounted for permanent
storage. In addition, the end-product can be made electron-dense with osmium
tetroxide.

5.2. The peroxidase anti-peroxidase method

A further development of the indirect technique has led to the exceedingly sensitive
double immunoglobulin bridge (Mason *et al.* 1969) and unlabelled antibody
enzyme or peroxidase anti-peroxidase (PAP) methods (see Sternberger 1979).

This technique involves yet a third layer which is a rabbit antibody to peroxidase,
coupled with peroxidase to make a very stable peroxidase anti-peroxidase complex.
The complex, composed of rabbit γ-globulin and peroxidase, acts as a third-layer
antigen and becomes bound to the unconjugated goat anti-rabbit γ-globulin of the
second layer. The second-layer goat anti-rabbit γ-globulin must be in excess with
respect to the first layer so that there is competition between the antibody molecules for the bound first-layer primary antibody. Thus only one combining site
of each of the second-layer antibody molecules is occupied by the primary antibody, now acting as an immunoglobulin antigen, and the second site is free to combine with the PAP complex, another immunoglobulin antigen (Figs. 2 (p. 11), 7,
and 8).

Advantages

This method results in 100 to 1000 times higher sensitivity since the peroxidase
molecule is not chemically conjugated to the anti IgG but immunologically bound,
and loses none of its enzyme activity. In addition, much more peroxidase ends up
on the site of reaction than in the indirect method. It also allows for much higher
dilution of the first antibody, thus eliminating many of the unwanted antibodies
and reducing non-specific staining, and is particularly specific since the PAP complex is highly purified and will react only with the anti-rabbit γ-globulin of the
second layer. It will not react with non-specifically attached antibodies which are
not themselves anti-IgG. It will not itself attach to tissue, provided that suitable

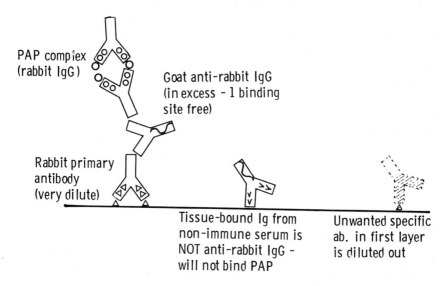

PAP complex
(rabbit IgG)

Goat anti-rabbit IgG
(in excess – 1 binding
site free)

Rabbit primary
antibody
(very dilute)

Tissue-bound Ig from
non-immune serum is
NOT anti-rabbit IgG –
will not bind PAP

Unwanted specific
ab. in first layer
is diluted out

Fig. 7. Unlabelled antibody-enzyme (peroxidase anti-peroxidase, PAP) method of Sternberger after blocking with non-immune serum from species in which second antibody was raised.

blocking with normal serum has been carried out, so background staining is minimal. It can also be usefully used at the ultrastructural level since the PAP complex has a characteristic appearance in the electron microscope and can be identified at the site of reaction and distinguished from non-specific electron density.

In all the bridge methods the immunostaining end-points may be intensified by repetition of staining sequences. (See Ordronneau *et al.* 1981 for a comparison of unlabelled antibody bridge techniques.)

Disadvantage

The disadvantage of the PAP technique is that it requires an extra reagent and adds a further step to the staining sequence.

Alternative enzyme labels

Another enzyme becoming widely used in immunocytochemistry is alkaline phosphatase (from calf intestine). It was originally introduced for quantitative work with the ELISA technique (see below) providing a soluble coloured end-product of reaction that could be measured with a spectrophotometer. However, the enzyme can also be reacted with an azo dye technique yielding a coloured precipitate, usually red or blue, suitable for immunocytochemistry. Alkaline phosphatase can

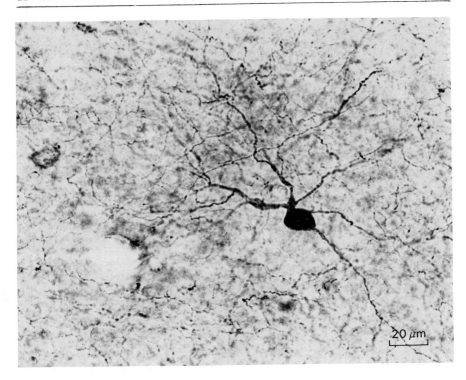

Fig. 8. Rat brain (piriform cortex) immunostained by the peroxidase anti-peroxidase method for neuropeptide Y (NPY). An immunoreactive cell body with dendrites is shown. NPY is a putative neurotransmitter. Tissue preparation. The rat brain was fixed by perfusion with 4 per cent p-formaldehyde in phosphate-buffered saline, then sectioned without freezing on a Vibratome. This 50 μm section was immunostained as a free-floating preparation. There is no counterstain.

be conjugated to the detecting antibody, or immunologically bound to a mono-clonal anti-alkaline phosphatase to give a stable, soluble complex similar to the PAP complex, although not cyclic, and used as a third layer in the same way as PAP (Mason and Sammons 1978; Mason *et al.* 1983; Cordell *et al.* 1984). Endogenous alkaline phosphatase may be a problem in fresh tissue, but the non-intestinal iso-enzymes can be inactivated by including 1mM levamisole in the development medium (Ponder and Wilkinson 1981). If fresh intestinal tissue is to be stained, this method is not suitable. The bright red or blue of the end-product of reaction is attractive and useful in double staining methods (see p. 24). A disadvantage is that the end-products of some development methods are partly or completely soluble in alcohol and preparations must be mounted in water-based media. One development method yields a solvent-fast red dye (Malik and Damon 1978).

   Glucose oxidase, another enzyme label, offers the advantage of being absent from animal tissues so that there is no need for a step to block endogenous enzyme (see Suffin *et al.* 1979).

Modifications of the basic methods

6.1. Double or multiple staining

It is often useful to be able to stain for two or more antigens in the same section. This can be achieved with peroxidase-conjugated antibodies developed with different couplers to produce differently coloured end-products (Nakane 1968). After development of the first immunostain with DAB, for example, the insoluble brown reaction product is deposited on the tissue section at the site of reaction. The deposit remains on the section while all the immune reagents (antibodies and PAP) that have taken part in the reaction, together with their peroxidase labels, are dissociated from the antigen in the tissue by a prolonged acid buffer rinse. A second antibody is then applied and the whole method is repeated using a different coupler, such as 4-chloro-1-naphthol (see § A.7), which gives a blue-coloured end-product (Fig. 9). Thus, for example, glucagon cells may be stained brown and insulin cells blue in the same pancreatic islet section (Colour Plate 2, inside back cover). It is also possible to add a third colour, red or green, according to the method chosen.

A green colour can be produced by o-dianisidine di–HCl (Colman *et al.* 1976) and red by 3-amino-9-ethyl carbazole (Colour Plate 3, inside back cover) or α-naphthol with pyronin (Nakane 1968).

The reason for dissociating the antibody between the two reactions is that unused peroxidase from the first reaction might react again in the second peroxidase reaction and also that, if the two primary antibodies are raised in the same animal, the primary antiserum number 2 might attach to any unused sites on the second-layer antibody of the first reaction. Careful controls are thus essential to make sure that the entire first antigen–antibody complex has been completely removed by the acid.

One problem of this method is that highly avid antibodies are difficult to disso-ciate, even in strong acid. Tramu's method may be more effective. Tramu *et al.* (1978) have introduced a slightly different double-staining method, less damaging to the tissue and other antigens, whereby the first immunostain is carried out by the 4-chloro-1-naphthol method. The section is then photographed and the antigen–antibody complex is dissociated by a short oxidation in acidified potassium per-manganate. The naphthol reaction product may then be dissolved in alcohol. Restaining, starting with the second antibody of the first reaction, should give a

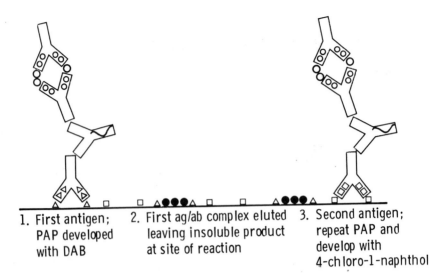

1. First antigen;
   PAP developed
   with DAB

2. First ag/ab complex eluted
   leaving insoluble product
   at site of reaction

3. Second antigen;
   repeat PAP and
   develop with
   4-chloro-1-naphthol

Fig. 9. Double immunoperoxidase labelling by PAP method after Nakane.

negative result, indicating that the complex has been entirely removed. The second stain is then carried out and the section is photographed. Photographs of the same area may be compared. If the naphthol stain is not dissolved, the two antigens may be seen simultaneously. It has been suggested (Sternberger and Joseph 1979) that under appropriate antibody concentration conditions, double immunostaining with primary antibodies raised in the same species can be successfully carried out without dissociation of the first reaction. This was confirmed by Valnes and Brandtzaeg (1982) who prefer, however, to use a mixture of separately labelled primary antibodies. A method of avoiding cross-over of antibodies while allowing sequential revelation of two antigens is that of Wang and Larsson (1985). After staining of the first antigen has been carried out hot formaldehyde vapour is used to block remaining immunoglobulin-combining sites before application of the second primary antibody.

Another technique that does not need an elution step is the double immuno-enzymatic method (Mason and Sammons 1978). This requires primary antibodies raised in different species and non-cross-reacting second antibodies. One set of reactions is labelled with alkaline phosphatase and the other with peroxidase. Except for the final enzyme development, the two methods are carried out simultaneously with a mixture of two reagents in each layer. Where rabbit PAP and mouse alkaline phosphatase anti-alkaline phosphatase (APAAP) complexes are available, the method can be shortened (Mason *et al.* 1983; Fig. 10, this volume; Colour Plate 4, inside back cover). A method for developing alkaline phosphatase is given in Appendix 9.

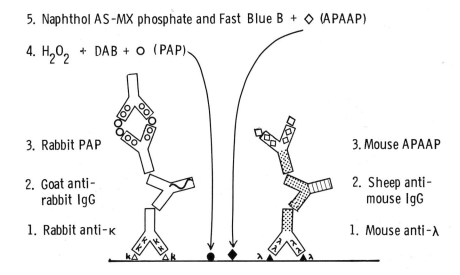

5. Naphthol AS-MX phosphate and Fast Blue B + ◇ (APAAP)

4. H_2O_2 + DAB + ○ (PAP)

3. Rabbit PAP

2. Goat anti-
   rabbit IgG

1. Rabbit anti-κ

3. Mouse APAAP

2. Sheep anti-
   mouse IgG

1. Mouse anti-λ

Fig. 10. Double staining by double immunoenzymatic method for κ and λ light chains (after Mason *et al.* 1983). Each layer consists of two immune reagents. Enzymes are developed separately. Kappa chains stain brown; lambda chains stain blue.

6.2. Labelled-antigen methods

A new approach to immunostaining, the radioimmunocytochemistry (RICH) technique, was introduced by Larsson and Schwartz (1977). A radioactive label (^{125}I) is attached to an antigen, say gastrin, which is then reacted with excess of anti-gastrin. The specific anti-gastrin molecules are thus radiolabelled with the antigen, but still have one binding site free for attachment to the tissue. The advantage of this one-step method is that only the specifically bound antibody will be detected in the subsequent autoradiograph. The disadvantages are that each antibody must be labelled individually, that the techniques of radiolabelling and autoradiography can be difficult and that the development of the reaction takes several days. Enzyme-labelled antigen was used similarly by Mason and Sammons (1979) and gold-labelled antigen by Larsson (1979) (Fig. 11).

6.3. Hapten-sandwich method

Another ingenious method for avoiding non-specific background staining is the hapten-sandwich technique using monoclonal anti-hapten antibodies as a bridge (Jasani *et al.* 1981). Nonspecific tissue binding sites are first blocked with non-

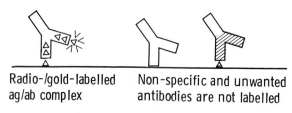

Radio-/gold-labelled   Non-specific and unwanted
ag/ab complex   antibodies are not labelled

Fig. 11. Labelled-antigen method.

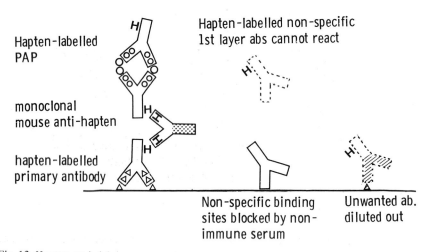

Hapten-labelled
PAP

Hapten-labelled non-specific
1st layer abs cannot react

monoclonal
mouse anti-hapten

hapten-labelled
primary antibody

Non-specific binding   Unwanted ab.
sites blocked by non-   diluted out
immune serum

Fig. 12. Hapten sandwich.

immune serum from the primary antibody donor. The primary antibody, labelled with a hapten (small antigen molecule) such as dinitrophenyl aminoproprionitrile imido ester, is the next layer, followed by a monoclonal antibody to the hapten and a hapten-labelled PAP complex, from any species, which is revealed by development of the peroxidase. Primary antigenic sites only are stained (Fig. 12).

6.4. Gold-labelling methods

Several recently developed methods rely on labelling with colloidal gold particles. These methods were originally introduced for electron microscopy (Faulk and

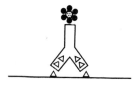

Fig. 13. Protein A/gold complex reacts with Fc portion of primary antibody.

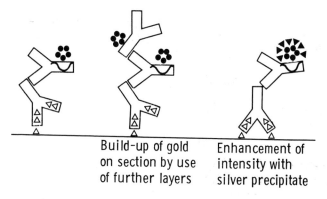

Build-up of gold
on section by use
of further layers

Enhancement of
intensity with
silver precipitate

Fig. 14. Gold-labelled antibody – indirect method.

Taylor 1971) as the gold particles are easily visible in the electron microscope, but they are also useful for light microscopy. In one method (Roth *et al.* 1978), advantage is taken of the ability of Protein A from the bacterium, *Staphylococcus aureus*, to bind to the Fc portion of immunoglobulins and to colloidal gold particles. A Protein A/gold complex is used as the second layer of the immunostain and at electron microscopical level, the attached gold particles may be seen over the site of reaction of the Protein A with the immunoglobulin first-layer antibody (Fig. 13).

This simple method is beginning to find great use in immunocytochemistry at the ultrastructural level. Its disadvantage is that it detects all available immunoglobulin in the section. Blocking steps with normal serum should be omitted in this technique. Protein A has also been conjugated with peroxidase and with ferritin.

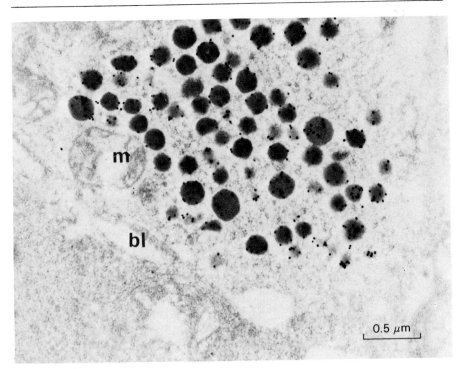

Fig. 15. Human colon. Electron micrograph showing secretory granules in an enteroglucagon endocrine cell immunostained by an indirect immunogold method using a rabbit antibody to glucagon followed by goat anti-rabbit IgG labelled with 20 nm diameter gold particles. Note that the gold particles are clustered over the secretory granules. Tissue preparation. The tissue was fixed in 2.5 per cent glutaraldehyde but was not post-fixed in osmium tetroxide. It was embedded in araldite and ultrathin sections were immunostained on-grid and counterstained with uranyl acetate and lead citrate. m, mitochondrion; bl, basal lamina.

Gold-labelled antigen detection (GLAD) has also been used (Larsson 1979) in the same way as in the RICH method (see Fig. 11) and gold particles have now been used to label second-layer antibody for an indirect staining technique, particularly at electron microscopial level (Romano *et al.* 1974; Horisberger 1979; De Mey *et al.* 1981, 1983; Figs. 14–16, this volume and see § A10).

One advantage of both these methods is that the gold complex has an intense red colour which can be seen in the light microscope. Thus, not only can the reactivity of the antibody or tissue be checked in the light microscope before electron microscopy is attempted, but the gold label can be used in double staining, providing a pleasing contrast to peroxidase visualization by the 4-chloro-1-naphthol (blue) or diaminobenzidine (brown) reaction products (Gu *et al.* 1981). Reduction of the gold particles by silver lactate to give an intense black colour greatly increases the sensitivity of the immunogold methods (Holgate *et al.* 1983a, b; Springall *et al.* 1984; Hacker *et al.* 1985; Fig. 14, Plate 6 this volume).

Since gold particles can be made in different sizes from 5 to 30 nm, it is possible

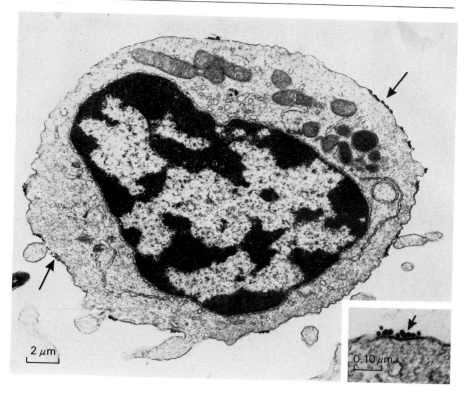

2 μm

0.10 μm

Fig. 16. Normal human blood T lymphocyte. Electron micrograph showing cell membrane marked with monoclonal antibody OKT 4 and rabbit anti-mouse IgG labelled with 20 nm diameter gold particles (arrows). OKT 4 positivity indicates that the cell belongs to the T-helper subset. Tissue preparation. The immunoreaction was carried out on unfixed blood cells. The cells were then fixed in 3 per cent glutaraldehyde followed by osmium tetroxide and embedded in araldite. Ultrathin sections were counterstained with uranyl acetate and lead citrate. Electron micrograph by courtesy of Dr D. Catovsky, Leukaemia Unit, Hammersmith Hospital, London.

to carry out multiple staining at the electron microscopical level, most easily by direct labelling of several first-layer antibodies with differently sized particles (Fig. 17). A 'cocktail' of labelled antibodies put on a section of duodenum could result in several cells containing different hormones, such as CCK, GIP, and secretin, being differentially labelled and demonstrated in one section. The indirect technique can also be used in double or triple staining if staining is carried out sequentially or with non-cross-reacting antibodies (Fig. 17) as in the double immunoenzymatic method. Bendayan (1982) has even stained different faces of the same grid with separate antibodies conjugated with differently sized gold particles. In addition, the presence of more than one immunoreactive antigen in the same granule or other organelle can be shown (Ravazzola and Orci 1980; Varndell *et al.* 1982).

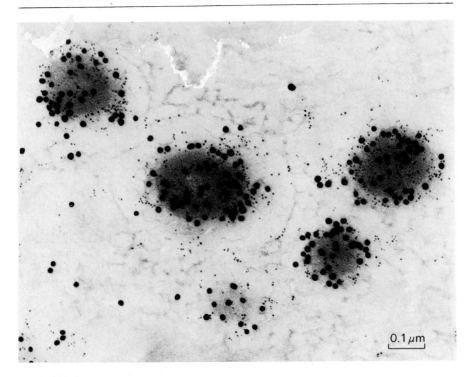

Fig. 17. Rat pancreatic islet cell. Electron micrograph showing double immunogold staining of insulin and C peptide. The ultrathin section was treated simultaneously with guinea pig anti-insulin and rabbit anti-C peptide (to demonstrate part of the insulin precursor molecule). The second layer was a 'cocktail' of goat anti-guinea pig IgG conjugated with 20 nm diameter gold particles and goat anti-rabbit IgG conjugated with 5 nm diameter gold particles. Note that the granules are marked by both labels. Tissue preparation. The tissue was freeze-dried at a very low temperature, fixed in osmium tetroxide vapour, and embedded in araldite. After the immunostain the section was counterstained with uranyl acetate and lead citrate. The tissue was prepared by Dr R.W. Dudek, University of East Carolina, North Carolina, USA.

These staining methods, as much as the well established peroxidase or fluorescence techniques, obviously depend on correct fixation and unmasking of the tissue antigen. The clarity with which gold labelling reveals antigen sites in the electron microscope has meant that they have largely superseded peroxidase and the semithin-thin comparison methods. For further reading see Polak and Varndell (1984).

6.5. Avidin—biotin methods

New labelling methods with great potential which are claimed to improve the sensitivity of immunostaining techniques and to avoid PAP, which is complicated

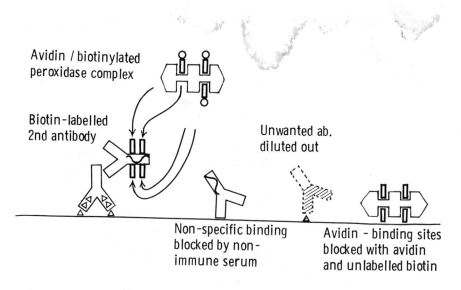

Fig. 18. Avidin–biotin complex (ABC) method.

to produce, involve the use of avidin and biotin. Avidin is a large glycoprotein from egg white which has a very high affinity (four binding sites per molecule) for biotin, a vitamin of low molecular weight found in egg yolk. Biotin can be coupled to antibody in a high molecular proportion, or to a label such as peroxidase. Avidin, too, may be labelled, for example with peroxidase or fluorescein. Consequently, these reagents may be used in a variety of immunostaining techniques. The one described below is the avidin–biotin complex (ABC) method. (For a full discussion of the methods and comparison with other techniques, see Guesdon *et al.* 1979; Hsu and Raine 1981; Hsu *et al.* 1981; Childs and Unabia 1982.)

The first layer is rabbit anti-antigen. The second layer is biotinylated goat anti-rabbit IgG. The third layer is a complex of avidin and biotinylated peroxidase which are reacted together in such proportion that some biotin-binding sites on the avidin molecule are not filled by biotinylated peroxidase, but are free to react with the biotin of the second layer antibody. The peroxidase is then developed by the DAB or any other technique (Fig. 18). It is thus obvious that a very large amount of peroxidase will be attached to each primary antigen site. These methods, too, may be used in electron microscopic immunocytochemistry using the usual variety of electron-dense labels.

A method of avoiding unwanted avidin binding to biotin which is widely distributed in tissues such as liver and kidney, has been described by Wood and Warnke (1981). The blocking takes the form of reacting the tissue with uncon-jugated avidin, which is then saturated with biotin. Because each biotin molecule has only one avidin-binding site, this procedure effectively blocks further non-specific attachment of the peroxidase-labelled avidin—biotin complex.

The substitution for avidin of streptavidin, derived from *Streptococcus avidini*, is a recent innovation. The streptavidin molecule is uncharged relative to animal tissue, unlike avidin which has an isoelectric point of 10, and therefore electrostatic binding to tissue is eliminated. In addition, streptavidin does not contain carbohydrate groups which might bind to tissue lectins. In other respects the molecule behaves in a similar way to avidin (Coggi *et al.* 1986).

7

Specificity problems and essential controls

In immunocytochemistry a positive-appearing result may well be genuine, but there are risks of non-specific reactions which must be eliminated before the result can be accepted (Tables 3 and 4).

Table 3. *Essential controls*

Method controls
1. Known positive control tissue included each time.
2. Test tissue stained
  a. with non-immume serum as first layer;
  b. with inappropriate antiserum as first layer;
  c. omitting first layer.
All these should be negative.

Antiserum specificity controls
3. Antibody (at maximum dilution compatible with good positive staining) pre-adsorbed with specific antigen (0.1–10 nmol/ml).

Should give negative stain.

4. Antibody at same dilution as in no. 3 pre-adsorbed with inappropriate antigen.

Should give positive stain.

5. Antibody at same dilution as in no. 3 adsorbed with antigen fragments or with structurally related antigen.

Result could help to determine the molecular structure of the substance being stained and the region-specificity of the antibody.

7.1. Non-specificity of antisera

This is due to

1. The heterogeneous population of antibodies in the donor's serum which may react with tissue components additional to the required specific antigen;

2. Shared amino-acid sequences between related substances particularly peptides, which may mean that a given antibody will react with several substances instead of just one.

7.2. Remedies for non-specificity due to heterogeneity of antibody

Immunoabsorption

The antisera can be 'purified' by immunoabsorption with the specific antigen bound to a solid phase such as sepharose beads; the antibody is subsequently eluted. However, it must be remembered that useful antibodies for immunocytochemistry are very avid and it will be difficult to elute such an antibody from the antigen used for absorption so that much of the antibody may be lost, and the eluted antibodies, although pure, will be of low avidity.

Dilution

High dilution of the antiserum results in diminution of the amount of unwanted antibody compared with the amount of wanted, specific antibody in the serum. The amount of unwanted specific binding may be reduced to the point where it becomes negligible.

Absorption with tissue powder, serum, or albumin

Non-specific attachment of immunoglobulins to tissue components by hydrophobic or electrostatic forces can be prevented by absorption of the antiserum with common tissue constituents such as albumin, or by a tissue powder (e.g. acetone-dried liver) from the species in which the staining is to be done. Alternatively, the tissue to be stained may be reacted first with albumin or with non-immune serum from the species donating the second-layer antibody. This occupies most of the non-specific tissue-binding sites, but the bonds are weaker than antigen–antibody reactions and allow the specific sites to react with the highly competitive primary antibody. One per cent of the normal serum may be added to the working dilution of the antibody. Attachment of immunoglobulin to Fc receptors in the tissue is not usually a problem after fixation, but may be confusing in unfixed tissue such as tissue cultures or suspensions of whole cells in which surface antigens are being investigated. The use of Fab fractions instead of whole immunoglobulin molecules should avoid the danger of this kind of unwanted staining.

Absorption with specific antigen

Control of staining by absorption of the antibody with its specific antigen prior to use should result in lack of staining. Absorption with other related or unrelated substances should have no effect. This is an essential negative control to be carried out with every new antiserum or new tissue site of reaction. It is also essential to include a known positively-reacting section in every test on experimental tissue as a method control to show that all the antibodies are in working order.

Absorption is best carried out on a solid-phase immunoadsorbent, such as sepharose beads coated with the antigen, which entirely removes the combining antibodies from the solution. In conventional liquid-phase absorption there is a possibility that soluble antigen—antibody complexes with antibodies of low avidity may dissociate, allowing the antibody to recombine with tissue antigen. In practice this is probably not a problem since antibodies which are useful for immunocytochemistry are, of necessity, highly avid, or they would not stay attached to the tissue antigen during the prolonged staining and washing steps. The disadvantage of the solid-phase absorbent is that the amount of antigen cannot be regulated easily. Comparison between different antisera is, therefore, difficult, whereas, in the liquid-phase absorption, it is possible to add a known amount of antigen, preferably calculated in nmol ml^{-1}, for comparison of absorption requirements of different antisera. The amount required to remove all staining from the antiserum can easily be titrated. 0.1 per cent bovine serum albumin should be added to the antibody diluent to prevent (by competition) the small quantity of antibody in the diluted solution from adhering unspecifically to the walls of the vial in which the absorption is carried out.

An ingenious way of checking the staining specificity if there is a shortage of enough pure antigen for absorption has been suggested by MacIver and Mepham (1982). It makes use of the competition for antigen in the tissue by antibodies raised in different species. For instance, when staining for IgG in human kidney with a rabbit anti-IgG, the section was exposed to a mixture of rabbit and goat antibodies to human IgG with goat anti-IgG in excess. The succeeding goat anti-rabbit IgG and rabbit PAP should give very much reduced staining on specific sites than with the rabbit anti-human IgG alone in the first layer. However, removal of staining by absorption with specific antigen remains the most satisfactory control.

7.3. Remedies for non-specificity due to cross-reactivity

Genuine cross-reactivity is impossible to eliminate. The only check is to use a variety of antibodies to different portions of the molecule if these are available.

Table 4. *Non-specific staining: problems and remedies*

Indirect immunofluorescence method

Problems	Remedies
High background fluorescence	1. Dilute primary and/or secondary antibody further. 2. Block with normal serum from donor species of second layer prior to staining with first layer. 3. Remove unbound fluorescein isothiocyanate from second layer on Sephadex G50 column. 4. Absorb primary and secondary antibodies with albumin or tissue powder from species to be stained.

Immunoperoxidase and PAP methods

Problems	Remedies
Background peroxidase or 'non-specific' staining of leukocytes, red blood cells.	1. Dilute primary and/or secondary antibody further. 2. Block with more concentrated (up to neat) normal serum from donor species of second layer before staining with primary antibody; block with normal serum between the first and second layers as well. Add detergent (Triton X-100, 0.2 per cent) to rinsing buffers or dilute the primary antibody in buffer of high ionic strength (add sodium chloride to 2.5%) (Grube 1980) to prevent non-specific attachment of protein. 3. Try stronger or longer or different peroxidase blocking technique. eg. 0.3 per cent H_2O_2 in buffer, methanol, or ethanol; sodium nitro-ferricyanide (1 per cent in methanol with 1 per cent acetic acid); periodate/borohydride. 4. Develop the peroxidase by the Hanker–Yates method, said to be specific for plant (i.e. horseradish) peroxidase and not to react with animal (tissue endogenous) peroxidase. 5. Absorb primary antiserum with albumin or tissue powder. 6. Affinity purification of primary antibody (but it may be of low avidity when eluted). 7. Remove complement from primary antibody by adding an unrelated antigen/antibody complex or by heating antiserum to 56°C for 30 mins. 8. Use an alkaline phosphatase system instead of a peroxidase system (block endogenous enzyme with 20 per cent acetic acid or add Levamisole to incubating medium (Ponder and Wilkinson 1981.)
Cross-reactivity of one antibody with several antigens.	1. Use of a variety of different antisera or region-specific antisera to the antigen you are interested in.

In vitro methods for testing antibodies and checking antigens

8.1. Enzyme-linked immunosorbent assay (ELISA)

This is not strictly immunocytochemistry, but is an *in vitro* method of testing for antibodies or antigens (Voller *et al.* 1976; O'Beirne and Cooper 1979).

When used for testing antibodies, say the first bleeding from a batch of 10 immunized rabbits, a known quantity of the antigen is applied to the inside surface of the cups of a microhaemagglutination plate. The second layer consists of the antisera to be tested in a series of dilutions and the third layer is a standard preparation of alkaline phosphatase-conjugated goat anti-rabbit immunoglobulin. The enzyme is then developed and the colour in each cup can be estimated by eye or read in a colorimeter. Positive and negative controls are, of course, included to provide a standard for each test. The second antibody may be radiolabelled and the results read in a scintillation counter.

ELISA is less sensitive than radioimmunoassay (see below), requiring somewhat lower dilutions of antibody approaching those used in immunocytochemistry and is less reliable than radioimmunoassay since the amount of peptide attached to the plastic cup and the type of binding sites left free are, at present, unpredictable. However, it more nearly resembles immunocytochemistry since it is the antibody and not the antigen which carries the label and, where there is no available radio-immunoassay, ELISA provides a good screening test for antibodies and can be used to check for cross-reactivity or contaminating antibodies. It could also be adapted to test for antigens in tissue extracts.

8.2. Radioimmunoassay

This is a separate *in vitro* method (Yalow and Berson 1959; for an introduction to the method see Self *et al.* 1976). It is mostly used for estimating the quantity of an antigen in blood or tissue extract and depends on the competition between a given quantity of a labelled antigen and the unlabelled antigen in the extract for a given quantity of specific antibody. The ratio between the bound and unbound antigen in the final solution gives a measure of the quantity present in the original extract. Note that here it is the antigen and not the antibody which carries the label and that the label is a radioactive element, usually iodine. The method can also be used for testing antibodies.

8.3. Electroblot techniques

To identify exactly with which tissue proteins an antibody is reacting, an extract of the tissue is subjected to electrophoresis on acrylamide gel. Because it is difficult to immunostain directly in the gel, the separated proteins are transferred to nitrocellulose paper by an electroblotting technique and the paper strip is then stained by the antibody and a PAP method as if it were a section of tissue. A parallel strip of electrophoresed tissue extract on acrylamide gel is stained to reveal the protein bands and matched up against the immunostained paper strip. (see De Mey 1983*a*).

Pure antigens may also be spotted onto suitable paper and stained by the antibody being tested. It must be remembered that antigens *in vitro* may behave differently from the way they do when bound in tissue.

Applicat... ...f immunocy...ochemistry

Immunocytochemistry is now one of the most widely used tools for research and diagnosis. Provided that clean antibodies of high specificity and avidity are available, the number of problems to which the method is applicable is unlimited. A few examples are given below.

9.1. Histopathological diagnosis

Immunocytochemical methods are being increasingly used in histopathological diagnosis as more antibodies become commercially available and with the arrival of the monoclonals. One of the major diagnostic fields is in lymphomas, which can be accurately subtyped with antibodies to immunoglobulin heavy and light chains, together with monoclonal antibodies to T and B cell types (Taylor 1980). Antibodies to markers for other types of tumour are widely used and are particularly useful for determining the origin of metastases. They include antibodies to thyroglobulin and calcitonin for diagnosis of thyroid tumours and prostatic acid phosphatase and prostate antigen for prostatic tumours. Other useful markers are not unique to one type of tumour and may be found in a variety of neoplasms and normal tissues. Their use lies mainly in differential diagnosis; for example, the absence ·of immunostaining for carcinoembryonic antigen would exclude the diagnosis of adenocarcinoma of the large bowel (in the presence of adequate positive controls and appropriate tissue preservation) while its presence would reinforce such a diagnosis made on other grounds. Two other monoclonal antibodies, to cytokeratin and to an antigen found on all leukocytes (leukocyte common antigen, LCA) provide a highly useful means of differentiating between carcinoma (cytokeratin positive, LCA negative) and lymphoma (cytokeratin negative, LCA positive), in a case where the origin of the tumour is in doubt (Gatter *et al* 1985). Liver tumours often contain α-1-fetoprotein, as do yolk sac tumours.

Factor VIII-related protein is used to mark growths of endothelial origin, neurone-specific enolase for neural or endocrine tumours, glial fibrillary acidic protein for glial tumours. Immunoglobulin type and localization is diagnostic in many kidney and skin disorders and circulating autoantibodies can be identified by staining normal tissue with the patient's serum in many other diseases. Microorganisms can be positively identified with appropriate antibodies. Endocrine tumours of the gastro-entero-pancreatic system and of the pituitary can be identified by immunocytochemistry with antibodies to a range of peptide hormones (Fig. 19). (For more detailed information and further references see Polak and Van Noorden 1983, 1986.)

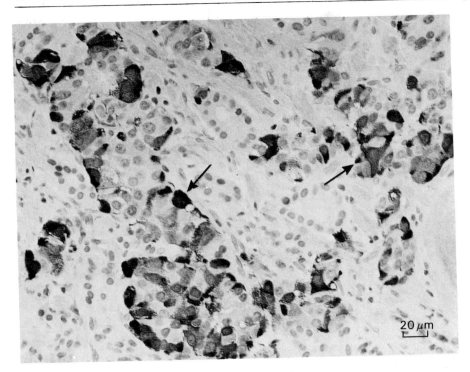

Fig. 19. Pancreatic endocrine tumour producing glucagon, immunostained by the peroxidase anti-peroxidase method. Note the proliferating glandular structures containing glucagon-positive cells (arrows). Tissue preparation: the tissue was fixed in Bouin's solution, then embedded in paraffin; 4 μm section, counterstained with haematoxylin.

9.2. Quantification

Quantification of immunocytochemical staining on a comparative basis can be carried out, given particular attention to standardization of methods, adequate sampling, and care in the selection of the parameters to be measured. A television image analyser can be used to give an indication of the volume density of an immunostained element compared with the rest of the tissue. For example, these techniques have recently shown that in some cases of neonatal hypoglycaemia there is not only a hyperplasia of insulin-producing cells in the pancreas, but also a significant reduction in the number of somatostatin cells, suggesting a deficiency in the normal inhibitory control exerted by somatostatin over insulin production (Polak and Bloom 1980). Quantification using three-dimensional computer mapping of immunostained material is a subject for the near future. For a general reference on quantification of tissue components see Aherne and Dunhill (1982).

A recently developed method of immunostaining slices of the mucosa and submucosa of the gut wall, freed from the muscle layer, as whole-mount preparations, has facilitated the estimation of the total population of particular endocrine cells in a sample (Ferri *et al.* 1982).

Comparative estimations of the amount of hormone per granule at the electron microscopical level may be possible with the gold- or ferritin-labelling techniques by counting the number of particles lying on a granule section (see Kraehenbuhl *et al.* 1980). To date, there is no way of estimating the absolute amount of an antigen in a tissue by immunocytochemistry but, with the additional information provided by radioimmunoassay of tissue and serum samples and by studies of the ultrastructure of the tissue, a fair idea of the secretory activity of the tissue and its rate of turnover can be obtained.

9.3. Basic research

The applications of immunocytochemistry to all kinds of research problems are too numerous to list here. Suffice it to say that the method can be combined with many other techniques, for example, autoradiography, histochemical staining, and biogenic amine identification by formaldehyde-induced fluorescence.

9.4. New imaging techniques

Immunocytochemistry will certainly remain a useful tool for localizing tissue sites of the increasing numbers of known antigens. No doubt, tissue preparation methods and antibody specificity will continue to be improved.

However, certain other, non-immunological, methods of specific marking are now used, sometimes in combination with immunocytochemistry. These new systems also use variously labelled probes to identify tissue constituents and include receptor localization, lectin histochemistry, and hybridization histochemistry.

The localization of radiolabelled hormones to their receptor sites by autoradiography is already well established (see, for example, Kuhar and Uhl 1979). With regard to receptor studies, immunocytochemical methods have already been used, sometimes even on fixed paraffin sections (e.g. Taylor *et al.* 1981), but, as there is some doubt as to whether fixation and embedding can preserve all receptor sites adequately (Salih *et al.* 1979), the use of cell suspensions (Goldsmith *et al.* 1979), cell cultures (e.g. Buckley and Burnstock 1986) or ultrathin frozen sections (Tokuyasu 1980, 1983; Willingham *et al.* 1980) will probably be the basis for further development of immunostaining for antigens bound to their receptors on the cell surface or after internalization; these investigations are in their early stages at present.

Lectin histochemistry is another non-antibody method of marking tissue components, using enzyme-, gold-, or fluorescent dye-labelled lectins. Lectins are plant or animal proteins that can attach to tissue carbohydrates (e.g. in glycoproteins) with a high degree of specificity according to the lectin and the carbohydrate group (Roth 1978; Ponder 1983; Leathem 1986). Since the carbohydrates may be characteristic of a particular tissue, lectin binding may have diagnostic significance. Tissue-bound lectins may be localized immunocytochemically like receptor-bound ligands.

Hybridization histochemistry is a rapidly advancing technique. It provides a very sensitive method of identifying the site of production of a cellular constituent rather than its storage site by employing radiolabelled recombinant DNA to localize its complementary messenger RNA (Pochet *et al.* 1981; Hudson *et al.* 1981). Hybridization histochemistry is used, for example, in the demonstration of oncogenes, the transformed growth-regulating genes that may promote tumour growth in some cases (Gastl *et al.* 1986). The combination of hybridization histochemistry and immunocytochemistry is beginning to answer questions about the production and storage sites of cell products and whether two or more may be synthesized in the same cell, simultaneously or sequentially (Roberts and Wilcox 1986).

Microscopy

Immunofluorescent preparations must be viewed with a microscope providing light of the correct wavelength to give maximum excitation of the fluorescent label. Immunoperoxidase or other visible immunostains can be seen in an ordinary light microscope, perhaps fitted with modifications for dark field, epipolarization, or Nomarski differential-interference contrast optics.

It is generally acknowledged that fluorescence is most efficiently seen by epi-illumination, in which the incident light passes through the objective lens, which thus acts as a condenser, and is focused on the specimen. Emitted light is passed back to the eye by the same route. Loss of illuminating energy by absorption of the incident light by the glass slide which carries the specimen is thus avoided. This epi-illumination method also allows for a combination of fluorescence and transmitted light or phase-contrast illumination so that parts of the specimen other than those immunofluorescently stained may be viewed at the same time as the fluorescence.

The light source for viewing immunofluorescence is usually a mercury vapour or xenon arc lamp and light of the wavelength providing for maximum excitation of the fluorophore passes through appropriate filters to the specimen. If both rhodamine and fluorescein are to be used, the microscope will have to be fitted with two sets of interchangeable filters. The red fluorescence of rhodamine cannot be seen at the same time as the green fluorescence of fluorescein because the wavelengths for maximum excitation differ (rhodamine, 530 nm; fluorescein, 495 nm). The same field in a preparation that has been double stained (e.g. T-lymphocytes labelled with rhodamine and B-lymphocytes labelled with fluorescein) can be observed first with one set of filters and then with the other. A double-exposure photograph can be taken which will show both the red and the green cells in the field, and any structures that are simultaneously labelled with both rhodamine and fluorescein will appear as a mixture of the two colours, a shade of orange. This situation might apply in the case of a serum antibody (autoantibody) being tested for activity against gastrin cells, for example, by simultaneous or sequential staining of a piece of antrum with the serum and with an antibody to gastrin (Scherbaum et al. 1983) or in the differentiation of one population of cells from another (Valnes and Brandtzaeg 1982).

Peroxidase, alkaline phosphatase, and other enzyme labels developed by any of the different colour-ways and colloidal gold can of course been seen with a standard transmitted-light microscope. In many cases, Nomarski differential-interference contrast optics can be very helpful in enhancing the effect of very lightly stained structures or very fine ones such as nerve fibres, since they show the stained area in raised or lowered relief against a flat background (Fig. 20).

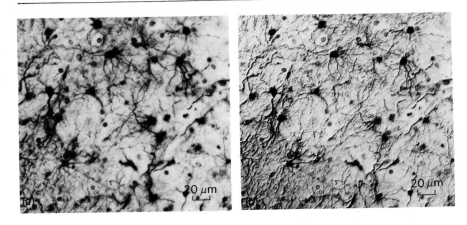

Fig. 20. Section of human brain showing normal astrocytes immunostained by the PAP method for glial fibrillary acidic protein. Note the enhancement in (b) of the fine fibres achieved with Nomarski interference-contrast optics. Tissue preparation: the tissue was fixed in formalin and embedded in paraffin. The section (6 μm) was treated with trypsin before being immunostained. Counterstained with haematoxylin.

If colloidal gold or silver are used as labels at the light microscopical level, the intensity of colour, particularly on thin (1 μm) sections, may be rather low under normal illuminating conditions. The use of dark-field illumination will enhance the effect considerably, the light being back-scattered by the metallic particles and making the object shine out. An even greater enhancement is achieved by epipolar illumination (De Mey 1983b).

Photomicrographs can be taken on any suitable film. *Kodak* technical pan 2415 is a useful film for high-contrast black and white photography. Fast films are preferred for fluorescence because the fluorescence fades exponentially on exposure to u.v. light. *Ilford* FP4 and HP5 are probably the most suitable films for black and white photography of fluorescence and Fujichrome 400D for colour photography of fluorescence.

For ordinary transmitted-light colour transparencies, using a 12 volt, 100 watt tungsten quartz light source, Ektachrome 50T is a suitable film, provided that Kodak colour compensating filters to CC25 (CC20 + CC5) are inserted in the light path.

Fluorescence preparations have the disadvantage that they are impermanent and should be photographed within a few days of preparation. Storage of slides in the dark will help to prevent fading, and addition of $25\,\text{g}\,\text{l}^{-1}$ of 1,4-diazobicyclo-(2-2-2)-octane to the mountant (Johnson *et al.* 1982) is also helpful in this respect. Water or glycerine immersion objectives may be used for high-power work.

Appendix: technical notes

The methods described here are in use in the author's laboratories. Many satis-factory variations of the methods are to be found in the literature.

A.1. Immunostaining by indirect method

Immunofluorescence

Paraffin sections

1. Remove wax and bring sections to water.
2. Remove mercury pigment if necessary with iodine and bleach in sodium thiosulphate.
3. Rinse sections in phosphate-buffered saline (PBS)*.
4. (Optional.) Block non-specific binding sites. Apply to sections a drop of normal serum from species supplying second antibody diluted 1/30 in PBS.
5. Do not rinse sections, but draw off excess serum with a tissue and/or (if blocking was not carried out) wipe slide except for area of section which should remain moist. Place the slides horizontally on a rack in a damp chamber, e.g. large petri dish containing some wet cotton wool or filter paper.
6. Apply to each section a drop of the primary antibody at a predetermined optimal dilution in PBS.
7. Incubate at $4°C$ (or room temperature) for 1 to 48 hours depending on the dilution of the antibody.
8. Rinse three times in PBS for five minutes each rinse.
9. Wipe slides dry except for the area of the section.
10. Apply a drop of fluorescein (or rhodamine)-conjugated antibody, e.g. goat anti-rabbit IgG, at a predetermined dilution in PBS for $\frac{1}{2}-1$ hour at room temperature.
11. Rinse 3 times in PBS.
12. Mount in PBS:glycerine, $1:9$ or $1:1$, (1,4-diazobicyclo-(2-2-2)-octane $25\,mg\,ml^{-1}$ may be added to the mounting medium to prevent fading (Johnson et al. 1982).

Cryostat sections

Method as above but see § A.3 for preparation

---

* 0.01 M phosphate-buffered normal saline, pH 7.0−7.2. Bovine serum albuʳ and sodium azide (0.01 per cent) are added to make diluent for primary aⁿ

Immunoperoxidase

Paraffin sections

1. Remove wax and bring sections to water.
2. Remove mercury pigment if necessary with iodine and bleach in sodium thiosulphate.
3. Rinse sections in phosphate-buffered saline (PBS).
4. Block endogenous peroxidase activity by soaking sections in 0.3 per cent hydrogen peroxide in PBS or water or methanol for 30 minutes.
5. Rinse in PBS.
6. Block non-specific binding sites with normal serum and apply first antibody as for immunofluorescence.
7. Rinse three times in PBS.
8. Apply peroxidase-conjugated second antibody diluted in PBS (no azide) for 30 minutes to one hour at room temperature.
9. Rinse three times in PBS.
10. Develop peroxidase by (modified) method of Graham and Karnovsky. Prepare solution just before use, and filter (optional). Incubating medium: 0.025– 0.05 per cent diaminobenzidine tetrahydrochloride (DAB)* in PBS with 0.015– 0.03 per cent H_2O_2. Sections may be incubated in drops of medium or immersed in a dish of solution. Incubation should be microscopically controlled and is usually adequate after five minutes at room temperature.
11. Rinse in water.
12. Counterstain nuclei with haematoxylin (lightly) or methyl green.
13. Dehydrate, clear, and mount.

Cryostat sections

Method as above, but see § A.3 for preparation.

A.2 Peroxidase anti-peroxidase (PAP) method

As for indirect immunoperoxidase, up to step 7. Dilution of primary antibody will generally be about 10 times higher for PAP method than for indirect method.

8. Apply unconjugated second antibody appropriately diluted in PBS for 30 minutes.
9. Rinse three times in PBS.
10. Apply PAP diluted in PBS (no azide) for 30 minutes.
11. Rinse three times in PBS.
12. Develop peroxidase as for indirect immunoperoxidase method.
13. Counterstain, dehydrate, clear, mount.

---

* Take care! It may be carcinogenic. See p. 19.

A.3. Cryostat sections

These are usually used for identification of surface antigens. Various treatments have been suggested.

1. Dry sections (about $5\,\mu m$) for 30 minutes at room temperature. Fix for 10 minutes in acetone or alcohol at room temperature or $4°C$. Rinse in PBS. Immunostain. (See Fig. 1 p. 6).

2. Dry sections at room temperature; then wrap in cling film or foil and put in $-20°C$ deep freeze with dessicant until used. Allow to warm up to room temperature before unwrapping, then fix in acetone or alcohol at room temperature or $4°C$, transfer to PBS with or without further drying, and immunostain.

3. Dry sections at room temperature for 30 minutes. Freeze-dry for 18 hours. Store, wrapped in foil at $-20°C$. Bring to room temperature. Fix in acetone or alcohol for 20 minutes at room temperature. Transfer to buffer without drying. Immunostain.

Examples of other recommended fixatives have included chloroform/acetone mixture, mixtures of formalin with acetone or ethanol, blocks pre-fixed with ethanol, formalin, or benzoquinone. Fixation will depend on antigen to be identified.

A.4. Intensification of the peroxidase reaction

1. Osmicate sections after development of the DAB in 1 per cent aqueous osmium tetroxide. Monitor darkness of reaction products with microscope. NB. Use osmium only in a fume cupboard.

2. Use a method of heavy-metal intensification. A useful one has been described by Hsu and Soban (1983). Add with stirring 2 ml of 1 per cent cobalt chloride to 100 ml of DAB solution. Incubate sections in this solution for five minutes before mixing in the appropriate amount of H_2O_2. The reaction product is dark blue-black (Colour Plate 5, inside back cover).

3. Add imidazole to the DAB reaction solution. The optimum pH for the peroxidase reaction is about 5.0, but although the sensitivity is increased at this pH the reaction product tends to diffuse from the site of production and also tends to crystallize. For these reasons the reaction is usually carried out at near neutral pH. Straus (1982) suggests the addition of 0.01 M imidazole to the DAB reaction solution to increase the rate and intensity of reaction. The imidazole solution is adjusted to the working pH with 1 N hydrochloric acid before addition.

A.5. Protease digestion

This is particularly useful for revealing 'over-fixed' antigenic sites in aldehyde-fixed paraffin sections. Semi-thin resin sections (resin removed) require a much shorter

ore dilute solution. After bringing sections to water, incubate them
s to one hour in, for example, 0.1 per cent trypsin (or pronase) in 0.1
um chloride (or buffer such as PBS) at $37°C$. The solution is brought
ith NaOH before use. A range of protease digestion times should be
g. 2, p. 11).

A.6. To prevent sections becoming detached from slides

Coat slides with poly-L-lysine (MW > 150 000; Sigma). This is particularly useful
where protease digestion is to be carried out, and for pre-fixed cryostat sections
of 'difficult' tissue.

Use clean glass slides, apply a very small drop (about $10 \mu l$) of poly-L-lysine
($1 \, \mathrm{mg \, ml^{-1}}$) at one end and spread over the slide with the end of another slide,
as for a blood film. A smooth layer, thin enough for interference colours to be
seen, should be achieved. It will dry almost at once. Batches of slides may be
prepared up to a week (at least) in advance of use. The coated slide should be
marked as the spread film is not visible. Vials of poly-L-lysine solution should be
stored frozen.

A.7. Peroxidase development by alternatives to DAB methods

Hanker's method (Hanker et al. 1977)

Hanker–Yates reagent*	75 mg
0.1 M Tris buffer, pH 7.6	
(or PBS)	100 ml
30 per cent H_2O_2	$100 \mu l$

Incubate sections until a dark blue/brown reaction product is obtained. Osmicate
if desired. Counterstain with neutral red or carmalum. Dehydrate, clear, and mount.

4-chloro-1-naphthol method (Nakane 1968)

4-chloro-1-naphthol	30–40 mg
dissolved in 100% alcohol	0.2–0.5 ml
Add with stirring 0.05 M Tris	
buffer pH 7.6 (or PBS)	100 ml
Add 30 per cent H_2O_2	$50–100 \mu l$
Filter (white precipitate) before use.	

A stronger stain is achieved by heating the incubating solution to about $50°C$,
filtering rapidly through coarse filter paper, and incubating the sections in the
hot filtrate (R. Buffa, personal communication).

Counterstain with carmalum.

* One part p-phenylene diamine HCL : 2 parts pyrocatechol (available from Polysciences or
Fluka).

Reaction product (dark blue) is soluble in alcohol, so mount in aqueous mountant (See Colour Plate 2, inside back cover).

Amino ethyl carbazole (AEC) method (Graham et al. 1965)

Soak sections in 0.05 M acetate buffer, pH 5.0. Incubate in the following solution.

AEC stock solution*	0.5 ml
0.05 M acetate buffer, pH 5.0	9.5 ml
30 per cent H_2O_2	10 μl

Filter on to sections and incubate for 5 to 10 minutes. Reaction product is red. Counterstain with haematoxylin. Reaction product is alcohol-soluble, so differentiate in aqueous acid and mount in an aqueous mountant (see Colour Plate 3, inside back cover).

A.8. Notes

1. Tris-buffered saline, 0.05 M, pH 7.6, may be used throughout instead of PBS.

2. Storage of DAB. A convenient way of storing DAB and avoiding unnecessary exposure to dust from the powder is to dissolve a 1 gram quantity (Sigma) in 40 ml of water and prepare 1 ml aliquots, each containing 0.025 g. The vials may then be frozen, and one vial contains sufficient DAB for 100 ml of incubating solution.

3. To 'decontaminate' glassware, etc. after use for DAB solutions, rinse with a little domestic bleach (sodium hypochlorite), to oxidize the DAB.

A. 9. Development of alkaline phosphatase to give a blue end-product

To 2 mg naphthol AS-MX phosphate dissolved in 0.2 ml dimethyl formamide (in glass vessel)

add

9.8 ml 0.1 M Tris/HC1 buffer, pH8.2.

This stock substrate solution may be stored at 4°C.

Just before use add Fast Blue B (or Fast Blue BB), 1 mg per ml, and filter on to the sections. Incubate at room temperature (or if necessary at 37°C) for 5–15 minutes, checking microscopically for bright blue reaction. Endogenous alkaline phosphatase may be blocked by adding 1 mM Levamisole to the incubating medium.

Stop the reaction by rinsing the preparations in water. Counterstain nuclei with Mayer's carmalum and mount in aqueous medium.

---

* Stock solution: 0.4 per cent 3-amino-9-ethylcarbazole in dimethylformamide.

A.10. Post-embedding electron microscopical immunocytochemistry using an indirect immunogold method

Tissue processing

1. Fix in standard glutaraldehyde or glutaraldehyde/formaldehyde fixative for two hours at 4°C, with or without additional osmium tetroxide fixation, depending on the antigen to be localized.

2. Dehydrate through graded alcohols and propylene oxide and embed in epoxy resin.

3. Cut 60–100 nm sections and collect them on cleaned, uncoated, 200–300 mesh, nickel or gold grids. Allow the sections to dry overnight.

Immunocytochemistry (see Fig. 15, p. 28)

It is convenient to carry out all incubations in multi-well microtest plates. Each well holds 15 μl of solution. It is preferable to microfilter all buffers and washing solutions (0.45 nm pore size). Thorough rinsing of the grids is best carried out by individual jet-washing from a syringe fitted with a microfilter or (when many grids are being stained) by placing the grids in a multiple grid holder suspended in a beaker of gently agitated washing buffer. The grids should not be allowed to dry during the staining process.

1. 'Etch' the sections in 10 per cent aqueous hydrogen peroxide to permeabilize the resin.

2. Wash in microfiltered distilled water.

3. Drain grids and incubate for 30 minutes at room temperature in drops of normal serum from the same species as the donor of the second antibody, diluted 1/30 in antiserum diluent (PBS containing 0.1 per cent bovine serum albumin (BSA) and 0.01 per cent sodium azide).

4. Drain the normal serum from the grids on to fibre-free absorbent paper and place the grids in the primary antibody, at optimal dilution (determined by experiment) in antibody diluent for one hour at room temperature to 48 hours at 4°C, depending on the antibody.

5. Wash thoroughly in 0.05 M Tris buffer, pH 7.2.

6. Wash thoroughly in 0.05 M Tris buffer, pH 7.2, containing 0.2 per cent BSA for three changes of 15 minutes each, with agitation.

7. Place grids in drops of 0.05 M Tris buffer, pH 8.2, containing 1 per cent BSA for five minutes.

8. Dilute the gold-labelled secondary antibody (e.g. goat anti-rabbit IgG)* at optimal dilution (determined by experiment) in 0.05 M Tris buffer, pH 8.2, containing 1 per cent BSA, and centrifuge it at 2000 g for 20 minutes to remove micro-aggregates of gold particles which accumulate on storage.

---

* Obtainable from Janssen Pharmaceutica. Antibodies may be conjugated with colloidal gold particles of several different diameters, e.g. 40 nm, 20 nm, 5 nm.

9. Incubate the grids in drops of the supernatant for one hour at room temperature.

10. Wash very thoroughly in large quantities of 0.05 M Tris buffer, pH 7.2, containing 0.2 per cent BSA, followed by Tris buffer, pH 7.2, without albumin, and distilled water.

11. Dry the grids by draining on fibre-free absorbent paper. Counterstain with uranyl acetate and lead citrate as for conventional electron microscopy.

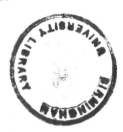

References

Aherne, W.A. and Dunhill, M.S. (1982). *Morphometry*. Edward Arnold, London.

Avrameas, S. and Uriel, J. (1966). Méthode de marquage d'antigènes et d'anticorps avec des enzymes et son application en immunodiffusion. *C. R. Acad. Sci., Paris, Ser. D* **262**, 2543–5.

Baskin, E.G., Erlandsen, S.L., and Parsons, J.A. (1979). Immunocytochemistry with osmium-fixed tissue. 1. Light microscope localizations of growth hormone and prolactin with the unlabeled antibody enzyme method. *J. Histochem. Cytochem.* **27**, 867–72.

Beauvillain, J.C. and Tramu, G. (1980). Immunocytochemical demonstration of LH-RH, somatostatin, and ACTH-like peptide in osmium-postfixed, resin-embedded median eminence. *J. Histochem. Cytochem.* **28**, 1014–17.

Bendayan, M. (1982). Double immunocytochemical labeling applying the protein A–gold technique. *J. Histochem Cytochem.* **30**, 81–5.

—— and Zollinger, M. (1982). Protein A–gold immunocytochemical labeling on osmicated tissues. *J. Histochem. Cytochem.* **30**, 576.

—— and —— (1983). Ultrastructural localization of antigenic sites on osmium-fixed tissue applying the protein A–gold technique. *J. Histochem. Cytochem.* **31**, 101–9.

Berod, A., Hartman, B.K., and Pujol, J.F. (1981). Importance of fixation in immunohistochemistry. *J. Histochem. Cytochem.* **29**, 844–50.

Bishop, A., Polak, J.M., Bloom, S.R., and Pearse, A.G.E. (1978). A new universal technique for the immunocytochemical localisation of peptidergic innervation. *J. Endocrinol.* **77**, 25P–26P.

Buckley, N.J. and Burnstock, G. (1986). Localisation of muscarinic receptors on cultured myenteric neurons: a combined autoradiographic and immunocyto chemical approach. *J. Neurosci.* **6**, 531–40.

Bullock, G. and Petrusz, P. (ed.) (1982). *Techniques in immunocytochemistry*, Vol. I. Academic Press, London.

—— and —— (ed.) (1983). *Techniques in immunocytochemistry*, Vol. II. Academic Press, London.

Bu'Lock, A., Vaillant, C., and Dockray, G.J. (1982). Immunohistochemical localisation of peptidergic nerve cell bodies in the gut following rational improvements to fixation with parabenzoquinone. *Reg. Peptides* **3**, 67.

Childs, G. and Unabia, G. (1982). Application of the avidin–biotin–peroxidase complex (ABC) method to the light microscopic localization of pituitary hormones. *J. Histochem. Cytochem.* **30**, 713–16.

Coggi, G., Dell'Orto, P., and Viale, G. (1986). Avidin-biotin methods. In *Immunocytochemistry, modern methods and applications*, (2nd edn), (ed. J.M. Polak and S. Van Noorden), pp. 54–70. John Wright & Sons, Bristol.

Colman, D.R., Scalia, F., and Cabrales, E. (1976). Light and electron microscopic observations on the anterograde transport of horseradish peroxidase in the optic pathway in the mouse and rat. *Brain Res.* **102**, 156–63.

Coons, A.H., Creech, H.J., and Jones, R.N. (1941). Immunological properties of an antibody containing a fluorescent group. *Proc. Soc. exp. Biol. Med.* **47**, 200–2.

———— and Kaplan, M.H. (1950). Localization of antigen in tissue cells. *J. exp. Med.* **91**, 1–13.

————, Leduc, E.H., and Connolly, J.M. (1955). Studies on antibody production. 1. A method for the histochemical demonstration of specific antibody and its application to a study of the hyperimmune rabbit. *J. exp. Med.* **102**, 49–59.

Cordell, J.L., Falini, B., Erber, W.N., Ghosh, A.K., Abdulaziz, Z., MacDonald, S., Pulford, K.A.F., Stein, H., and Mason, D.Y. (1984). Immunoenzymatic labeling of monoclonal antibodies using immune complexes of alkaline phosphatase and monoclonal anti-alkaline phosphatase (APAAP complexes). *J. Histochem. Cytochem.* **32**, 219–22.

Cuello, A.C., Priestley, J.V., and Milstein, C. (1982). Immunocytochemistry with internally labeled monclonal antibodies. *Proc. Natl. Acad. Sci. USA.* **79**, 665–9.

De Mey, J. (1983*a*). Raising and testing antibodies. In *Immunocytochemistry, practical applications in pathology and biology* (ed. J.M. Polak and S. Van Noorden), pp. 43–52. John Wright & Sons, Bristol.

———— (1983*b*). Colloidal gold probes in immunocytochemistry. In *Immunocytochemistry, practical applications in pathology and biology* (ed. J.M. Polak and S. Van Noorden), pp. 82–112. John Wright & Sons, Bristol.

————, Moeremans, M., Gevens, G., Nuydens, R., and De Brabander, M. (1981). High resolution light and electron microscopic localization of tubulin with the IGS (Immunogold Staining) method. *Cell Biol. int. Rep.* **5**, 889–99.

Elde, R., Hökfelt, T., Johansson, O., and Terenius, L. (1976). Immunohistochemical studies using antibodies to leucine–enkephalin: initial observations on the nervous system of the rat. *Neuroscience* **1**, 349–51.

Faulk, W.R. and Taylor, G.M. (1971). An immunocolloid method for the electron microscope. *Immunochemistry* **8**, 1081–3.

Ferri, G.-L., Harris, A., Wright, N.A., Bloom, S.R., and Polak, J.M. (1982). Quantification of endocrine cells in whole intestinal crypts and villi. *Histochem. J.* **14**, 692–5.

Finley, J.C.W. and Petrusz, P. (1982). The use of proteolytic enzymes for improved localization of tissue antigens with immunocytochemistry. in *Techniques in immunocytochemistry* (ed. G.R. Bullock and P. Petrusz), Vol. 1, pp. 239–49. Academic Press, London.

Gastl, G., Ward, J.M., and Rapp, U.R. (1986). Immunocytochemistry of oncogenes. In *Immunocytochemistry, modern methods and applications*, (2nd edn), (ed. J.M. Polak and S. Van Noorden), pp. 275–83. John Wright & Sons, Bristol.

Gatter, K.C., Heryet, A., Alcock, C., and Mason, D.Y. (1985). Clinical importance of analysing malignant tumours of uncertain origin with immunohistological techniques. *Lancet* i, 1302–5.

Goldsmith, P.C., Cronin, M.J., and Weiner, R.I. (1979). Dopamine receptor sites in the anterior pituitary. *J. Histochem. Cytochem.* **27**, 1205–7.

Graham, R.C. and Karnovsky, M.J. (1966). The early stages of absorption of injected horseradish peroxidase in the proximal tubules of mouse kidney: ultrastructural cytochemistry by a new technique. *J. Histochem. Cytochem.* **14**, 291–302.

——, Ludholm, U., and Karnovsky, M.J. (1965). Cytochemical demonstration of peroxidase activity with 3-amino-9-ethylcarbazole. *J. Histochem. Cytochem.* **13**, 150–2.

Grube, D., (1980). Immunoreactivities of gastrin (G) cells. II, Nonspecific binding of immunoglobulins to G-cells by ionic interactions. *Histochemistry,* **66**, 149–67.

Gu, J., de Mey, J., Moeremans, M., and Polak, J.M. (1981). Sequential use of the PAP and immunogold methods for the light microscopical double staining of tissue antigens. Its application to the study of regulatory peptides in the gut. *Reg. Peptides* **1**, 365–74.

Guesdon, J.L., Ternynck, T., and Avrameas, S. (1979). The use of avidin–biotin interaction in immunoenzymatic techniques. *J. Histochem. Cytochem.* **27**, 1131–39.

Hacker, G.W., Springall, D.R., Van Noorden, S., Bishop, A.E., Grimelius, L., and Polak, J.M. (1985). The immunogold-silver staining method. A powerful tool in histopathology. *Virchows Arch.* **406**, 449–61.

Hanker, J.S., Yates, P.E., Metz., C.B., and Rustioni, A. (1977). A new specific, sensitive and non-carcinogenic reagent for the demonstration of horseradish peroxidase. *Histochem. J.* **9**, 789–92.

Heyderman, E. (1979). Immunoperoxidase techniques in histopathology: applications, methods and controls. *J. clin. Pathol.* **32**, 971–8.

Holgate, C.S., Jackson, P., Cowen, P.N., and Bird, C.C. (1983*a*). Immunogold–silver staining – new method of immunostaining with enhanced sensitivity. *J. Histochem. Cytochem.* **31**, 938–44.

——, ——, Lauder, I., Cowen, P.N., and Bird, C.C. (1983*b*). Surface membrane staining of immunoglobulins in paraffin sections of non-Hodgkin's lymphomas using an immunogold–silver technique. *J. clin. Pathol.* **36**, 742–6.

Horisberger, M. (1979). Evaluation of colloidal gold as a cytochemical marker for transmission and scanning electron microscopy. *Biol. Cellulaire* **36**, 253–8.

Hsu, S.-M. and Raine, L. (1981). Protein A, avidin and biotin in immunocytochemistry. *J. Histochem. Cytochem.* **29**, 1349–53.

——, ——, and Fanger, H. (1981). Use of avidin–biotin–peroxidase complex (ABC) in immunoperoxidase techniques. *J. Histochem. Cytochem.* **29**, 577–80.

—— and Soban, E. (1982). Colour modification of diaminobenzidine (DAB) precipitation by metallic ions and its application to double immunohistochemistry. *J. Histochem. Cytochem.* **30**, 1079–82.

Huang, S. Minassian, H., and More, J.D. (1976). Application of immunofluorescent staining in paraffin sections improved by trypsin digestion. *Lab. Invest.* **35**, 383–91.

Huang, W.M., Gibson, S., Facer, P., Gu, J., and Polak, J.M. (1983). Improved section adhesion for immunocytochemistry using high molecular weight polymers of L-lysine as a slide coating. *Histochemistry* **77**, 275–9.

Hudson, P., Penschow, J., Shine, J., Ryan, G., Niall, H., and Coghlan, J. (1981). Hybridization histochemistry: use of recombinant DNA as a "homing probe" for tissue localization of specific mRNA populations. *Endocrinology* **108**, 353–6.

Hunt, S.P., Allanson, J., and Mantyh, P.W. (1986). Radioimmunocytochemistry. In *Immunocytochemistry, modern methods and applications,* (2nd edn), (ed. J.M. Polak and S. Van Noorden), pp. 99–114. John Wright & Sons, Bristol.

Husain, O.A.N., Millett, J.A., and Granger, J.M. (1980). Use of polylysine coated slides in the preparation of samples for diagnostic cytology with special reference to urine samples. *Clin. Pathol.* **33**, 309–11.

International Agency for Research on Cancer (1972). *Some inorganic substances, chlorinated hydrocarbons, aromatic amines, N-nitroso compounds and natural products,* Monograph 1, pp. 80–6. Monographs on the Evaluation of the Carcinogenic Risk of Chemicals to Humans, Lyon, France

Jasani, B., Wynford Thomas, D., and Williams, E.D. (1981). Use of monoclonal antihapten antibodies for immunolocalisation of tissue antigens. *J. clin. Pathol.* **34**, 1000–2.

Johnson, G.D., Davidson, R.S., McNamee, K.C., Russell, G., Goodwin, D., and Holborow, E.J. (1982). Fading of immunofluorescence during microscopy: a study of the phenomenon and its remedy. *J. Immunol. Methods* **55**, 231–42.

Johnstone, A. and Thorpe, R. (1982). *Immunochemistry in practice.* Blackwell, Oxford.

Kraehenbuhl, J.P., Racine, L., and Griffiths, G.W. (1980). Attempts to quantitate immunocytochemistry at the electron microscope level. *Histochem. J.* **12**, 317–32.

Kuhar, M.J. and Uhl, G.R. (1979). Histochemical localization of opiate receptors and the enkephalins. In *Neurochemical mechanisms of opiates and endorphins* (ed. H.H. Loh and D.H. Ross), pp. 53–68. Raven Press, New York.

Kung, P.C., Goldstein, G., Reinherz, E.L., and Schlossman, S.F. (1979). Monoclonal antibodies defining distinctive human T cell surface antigens. *Science* **206**, 348–9.

Larsson, L.-I. (1979). Simultaneous ultrastructural demonstration of multiple peptides in endocrine cells by a novel immunocytochemical method. *Nature* **282**, 743–5.

—— (1980). Problems and pitfalls in immunocytochemistry of gut peptides. In *Gastrointestinal hormones* (ed. G.B. Jerzy Glass), pp. 53–70. Raven Press, New York.

—— (1981). Peptide immunocytochemistry. *Prog. Histochem. Cytochem.* **13** (4).

—— and Schwartz, T.W. (1977). Radioimmunocytochemistry – a novel immunocytochemical principle. *J. Histochem. Cytochem.* **25**, 1140–8.

Leathem, A. (1986). Lectin histochemistry. In *Immunocytochemistry, modern methods and applications.* (2nd edn), (ed. J.M. Polak and S. Van Noorden) pp. 167–87. John Wright & Sons, Bristol.

MacIver, A.G. and Mepham, B.L. (1982). Immunoperoxidase techniques in human renal biopsy. *Histopathology* **6**, 249–67.

Malik, D.Y. and Damon, M.E. (1978). Improved double immunoenzymatic labelling using alkaline phosphatase and horseradish peroxidase. *J. Clin. Pathol.* **35**, 1092–4.

Mason, D.Y., Abdulaziz, Z., Falini, B., and Stein, H. (1983). Double immunoenzymatic labelling. In *Immunocytochemistry, practical applications in pathology and biology* (ed. J.M. Polak and S. Van Noorden), pp. 113–28. John Wright & Sons, Bristol.

—— and Sammons, R.E. (1978). Alkaline phosphatase and peroxidase for double immunoenzymatic labelling of cellular constituents. *J. clin. Pathol.* **31**, 454–60.

—— and —— (1979). The labeled antigen method of immunoenzymatic staining. *J. Histochem. Cytochem.* **27**, 832–40.

Mason, T.C., Phifer, R.F., Spicer, S.S., Swallow, R.A., and Dreskin, R.B. (1969).

An immunoglobulin–enzyme bridge method for localizing tissue antigens. *J. Histochem. Cytochem.* **17**, 563–9.

McLean, I.W. and Nakane, P.K. (1974). Periodate–lysine–paraformaldehyde fixative. A new fixative for immunoelectron microscopy. *J. Histochem. Cytochem.* **22**, 1077–83.

McMichael, A.J. and Fabre, J.W. (Eds.) (1982). *Monoclonal antibodies in clinical medicine.* Academic Press, London.

Milstein, C. (1980). Monoclonal antibodies. *Sci. Amer.* **243**, 56–64.

———, Galfre, G., Secher, D.S., and Springer, T. (1979). Monoclonal antibodies and cell surface antigens. *Cell Biol. int. Rep.* **3**, 1–16.

Nakane, P.K. (1968). Simultaneous localization of multiple tissue antigens using the peroxidase-labeled antibody method: a study on pituitary gland of the rat. *J. Histochem. Cytochem.* **16**, 557–60.

——— and Pierce, G.B. Jr. (1966). Enzyme-labeled antibodies: preparation and application for the localization of antigens. *J. Histochem. Cytochem.* **14**, 929–31.

O'Beirne, A.J. and Cooper, H.R. (1979). Heterogeneous enzyme immunoassay. *J. Histochem. Cytochem.* **27**, 1148–62.

Ordronneau, P., Lindstrom, P.B.M., and Petrusz, P. (1981). Four unlabeled antibody bridge techniques: a comparison. *J. Histochem. Cytochem.* **29**, 1397–404.

Pearse, A.G.E. and Polak, J.M. (1975). Bifunctional reagents as vapour and liquid phase fixatives for immunohistochemistry. *Histochem. J.* **7**, 179–86.

Pochet, R., Brocas, H., Vassart, G., Toubeau, G., Seo, H., Refetoff, S., Dumont, J.E., and Pasteels, J.L. (1981). Radioautographic localization of prolactin messenger RNA on histological sections by in situ hybridization. *Brain Res.* **211**, 433–8.

Polak, J.M. and Bloom, S.R. (1980). Decrease of somatostatin content in persistent neonatal hyperinsulinaemic hypoglycaemia. In *Current views on hypoglycaemia and glucagon* (ed. D. Andreani, P.J. Lefèbvre, and V. Marks), pp. 367–98. Academic Press, London.

——— and Van Noorden S. (Eds.) (1983). *Immunocytochemistry, practical applications in pathology and biology.* John Wright & Sons, Bristol.

——— and Van Noorden S. (ed.) (1983). *Immunocytochemistry, practical appli- and applications*, (2nd. edn). John Wright & Sons, Bristol.

——— and Varndell, I.M. (ed.) (1984). *Immunolabelling for electron microscopy.* Elsevier Scientific Publications, Amsterdam.

Ponder, B.A.J. (1983). Lectin histochemistry. In *Immunocytochemistry, practical applications in pathology and biology* (ed. J.M. Polak and S. Van Noorden), pp. 129–42. John Wright & Sons, Bristol.

——— and Wilkinson, M.M. (1981). Inhibition of endogenous tissue alkaline phosphatase with the use of alkaline phosphatase conjugates in immunohistochemistry. *J. Histochem. Cytochem.* **29**, 981–4.

Ravazzola, M. and Orci, L. (1980). A pancreatic polypeptide (PP)-like immunoreactant is present in the glicentin-containing cells of the cat intestine. *Histochemistry* **67**, 221–4.

Ritter, M.A. (1986). Raising and testing monoclonal antibodies for immunocytochemistry. In *Immunocytochemistry, modern methods and applications* (2nd edn) (ed. J.M. Polak and S. Van Noorden), pp. 13–25. John Wright & Sons, Bristol.

Roberts, J.L. and Wilcox, J.N. (1986). Hybridization histochemistry: analysis of specific mRNAs in individual cells. In *Immunocytochemistry, modern methods and applications*, (2nd edn), (ed. J.M. Polak and S. Van Noorden), pp. 199–204. John Wright & Sons, Bristol.

Roitt, I.M. (1980). *Essential immunology* (4th edn). Blackwell Scientific Publications, Oxford.

Romano, E.L., Sfolinski, C., and Hughes-Jones, N.S. (1974). An antiglobulin reagent labelled with colloidal gold for use in electron microscopy. *Immunochemistry* 11, 521–2.

Roth, J. (1978). The lectins – molecular probes in cell biology and membrane research. *Exp. Path. Suppl.* 3.

——, Bendayan, M., and Orci, L. (1978). Ultrastructural localization of intracellular antigen by the use of the Protein A–gold complex. *J. Histochem. Cytochem.* 26, 1074–81.

Salih, H., Murthy, G.S., and Friesen, H.G. (1979). Stability of hormone receptors with fixation: implications for immunocytochemical localization of receptors. *Endocrinology* 105, 21–6.

Scherbaum, W.A., Mirakian, R., Pujol-Borrell, R., Dean, B.M., Bottazzo, G.F. (1983). Indirect immunofluorescence in the study and diagnosis of organ-specific autoimmune diseases. In *Immunocytochemistry, practical applications in pathology and biology* (ed. J.M. Polak and S. Van Noorden) pp. 346–61. John Wright and Sons, Bristol.

Self, M., Rees, L.H., and Landon, J. (1976). An introduction to radioimmunoassay. *Med. Lab. Sci.* 33, 221–8.

Singer, S.J. and Schick, A.F. (1961). The properties of specific stains for electron microscopy prepared by conjugation of antibody molecules with ferritin. *J. Biophys. Biochem. Cytol.* 9, 519–37.

Springall, D.R., Hacker, G.W., Grimelius, L., and Polak, J.M. (1984). The potential of the immunogold-silver staining method for paraffin sections. *Histochemistry*, 81, 362–8.

Sternberger, L.A. (1979). *Immunocytochemistry* 2nd ed. John Wiley & Sons, New York.

—— (1983). Introduction, with emphasis on brain immunocytochemistry. In *Immunocytochemistry, practical applications in pathology and biology* (ed. J.M. Polak and S. Van Noorden), pp. 1–10. John Wright & Sons, Bristol.

—— and Joseph, F.A. (1979). The unlabeled antibody method. Contrasting color staining of paired pituitary hormones without antibody removal. *J. Histochem. Cytochem.* 29, 1424–9.

Straus, W. (1971). Inhibition of peroxidase by methanol and by methanol-nitroferricyanide for use in immunoperoxidase procedures. *J. Histochem. Cytochem.* 10, 682–8.

—— (1972). Phenylhydrazine as inhibitor of horseradish peroxidase for use in immunoperoxidase procedures. *J. Histochem. Cytochem.* 20, 949–51.

—— (1982). Imidazole increases the sensitivity of the cytochemical reaction for peroxidase with diaminobenzidine at a neutral pH. *J. Histochem. Cytochem.* 30, 491–3.

Suffin, S.C., Muck, K.B., Young, J.C., Lewin, K., and Porter, D.D. (1979). Improvement of the glucose oxidase immunoenzyme technic. *Am. J. clin. Pathol.* 71, 492–6.

Szelke, M. (1983). Raising antibodies to small peptides. In *Immunocytochemistry, applications in pathology and biology* (ed. J.M. Polak and S. Van Noorden), pp. 53–68. John Wright & Sons, Bristol.

Taylor, C.R. (1980). Immunohistologic studies of lymphoma: past, present and future. *J. Histochem. Cytochem.* **28**, 777–87.

——, Cooper, C.L., Kurman, R.J., Goebelsman, U., and Markland, F.S. (1981) Detection of estrogen receptor in breast and endometrial carcinoma by the immunocytochemical technique. *Cancer* **47**, 2634–40.

Tokuyasu, K.T. (1980). Immunochemistry on ultrathin frozen sections. *Histochem. J.* **12**, 381–403.

—— (1983). Present state of immunocryoultramicrotomy. *J. Histochem. Cytochem.* **31**, 164–7.

Tramu, G., Pillez, A., and Leonardelli, J. (1978). An efficient method of antibody elution for the successive or simultaneous localization of two antigens by immunocytochemistry. *J. Histochem. Cytochem.* **26**, 322–4.

Tubbs, R.R. and Sheibani, K. (1982). Chromogens for immunohistochemistry. *Arch. Pathol. Lab. Med.* **106**, 205.

Valnes, K. and Brandtzaeg, P. (1982). Comparison of paired immunofluorescence and paired immunoenzyme staining methods based on primary antisera from the same species. *J. Histochem. Cytochem.* **30**, 518–24.

Varndell, I.M., Tapia, F.J., De Mey, J., Rush, R.A., Bloom, S.R., and Polak, J.M. (1982) Electron-immunocytochemical localization of enkephalin-like material in catecholamine-containing cells of the carotid body, the adrenal medulla, and in pheochromocytomas of man and other mammals. *J. Histochem. Cytochem.* **30**, 682–90.

Voller, A., Bidwell, D., and Bartlett, A. (1976). Microplate enzyme immunoassays for the immunodiagnosis of virus infections. In *Manual of clinical immunology* (ed. N.R. Rose and H. Friedman) Chapter 69. American Society for Microbiology, Washington.

Wang, B. and Larsson, L.-I. (1985). Simultaneous demonstration of multiple antigens by indirect immunofluorescence and immunogold staining. *Histochemistry*, **83**, 47–56.

Weisburger, E.K., Russfield, A.B., Homburger, F., Weisburger, J.H., Boger, E., Van Dongen, C.G., Chu, K.C. (1978). Testing of twenty-one environmental aromatic amines or derivatives for long-term toxicity or carcinogenicity. *J. Environ. Pathol. Toxicol.* **2**, 325–56.

Wick, G., Traill, K.N., and Schauenstein, K. (ed.) (1982). *Immunofluorescence technology. Selected theoretical and clinical aspects.* Elsevier Biomedical Press, Amsterdam.

Willingham, M.C. (1980). Electron microscopic immunocytochemical localization of intracellular antigens in cultured cells: the EGS and ferritin bridge procedures. *Histochem. J.* **12**, 419–34.

——, Maxfield, F.R., Pastan, I. (1980) Receptor-mediated endocytosis of $alpha_2$-macroglobulin in cultured fibroblasts. *J. Histochem. Cytochem.* **28**, 818–23.

Wood, G.S. and Warnke, R. (1981). Suppression of endogenous avidin-binding activity in tissues and its relevance to biotin–avidin detection systems. *J. Histochem. Cytochem.* **29**, 1196–204.

Yalow, R.S. and Berson, S.A. (1959). Assay of plasma insulin in human subjects by immunological methods. *Nature* **184**, 1648–9.

Index

adherence of sections, 12, 48
alkaline phosphatase, 1, 21
    development, 49
alkaline phosphatase anti-alkaline phosphatase, 24
3-amino-9-ethylcarbazole, 20, 23, 49
antibody
    affinity, 6
    avidity, 6
    characteristics, 6
    monoclonal, 5
    penetration, 9
    production, 3
    region-specific, 4
    specificity, 33
    testing
        electroblot technique, 38
        ELISA, 37
        radioimmunoassay, 37
        titration, 13
    titre, 7
antigen
    availability, 8
    cell membrane, 6, 9, 29, 47
applications of immunocytochemistry
    histopathological diagnosis, 39
avidin-biotin methods, 30

background staining, 36
    remedies, 36

cell membrane antigens, 6, 9, 29, 47
4-chloro-1-naphthol, 23, 48
colloidal gold
    labelling, 26, 27, 28, 29, 50
    multiple staining, 28, 29, 30
controls, 33, 34
counterstains, 12
cryostat sections, 6, 8, 9, 10, 45, 46, 47

diaminobenzidine
    alternative reagents, 20, 48
    development of peroxidase, 46
    possible carcinogenicity, 19

direct method, immunofluorescence, 14, 15
double staining, 23
    with dissociation of first reaction, 23
    without dissociation of first reaction, 24
    double immunoenzymatic technique, 24, 25
    immunogold for electron microscopy, 26, 27, 28, 29, 30

electroblot technique, 38
electron-dense labels
    colloidal gold, 26, 27, 28, 29, 30, 50
    ferritin, 1
electron microscopical immunocytochemistry, 50
ELISA, 4, 37
endogenous peroxidase
    blocking methods, 19, 46
enhancement of reactions, 12, 21, 47
enzyme labels
    alkaline phosphatase, 1, 12, 21, 24
    glucose oxidase, 1, 22
    peroxidase, 1, 12, 19

fixation, 8, 9
    p-benzoquinone, 8, 9
    cross-linking reagents, 8
    diethyl pyrocarbonate, 8
    formaldehyde, 8, 9
    freeze-drying, 8
    periodate–lysine–paraformaldehyde, 9, 10
fluorescent labels
    fluorescein isothiocyanate, 1, 12
    rhodamine isothiocyanate, 1, 12

glucose oxidase, 1, 22

Hanker–Yates reagent, 20, 48
hapten sandwich method, 25, 26
histopathology, 39
hybridization histochemistry, 42

imidazole, 47

immunization, 3
    carrier protein, 3
immunofluorescence
    direct method, 14, 15
    indirect method, 14, 16, 17, 18, 45
immunogold method, 50
immunoperoxidase method, 46
indirect method
    advantages, 14
    immunoenzyme, 19, 46
        advantages, 19
        disadvantages, 19
        immunofluorescence, 14, 16, 17, 45
        immunogold, 27, 28, 50
        with silver intensification, 28

labelled antigen method, 25, 26
    gold, 28
    radioactive, 25
labelling procedure, 13
labels
    alkaline phosphatase, 1, 21, 24
    biotin, 1, 30
    colloidal gold, 1, 26, 27, 28, 29, 30
    electron-dense, 1
    enzyme, 1, 12
    fluorescent, 1, 12
    glucose oxidase, 1, 22
    hapten, 1, 25
    peroxidase, 1, 13, 19
    radioactive, 1, 13, 25
lectin histochemistry, 41

microscopy, 43
monoclonal antibodies, 5

Nomarski differential interference contrast
            optics (*or* Nomarski optics), 43, 44
non-specificity, 33, 36
    control absorption with antigen, 34
    cross-reactivity, 35, 37

remedies, 36
    absorption with tissue powder, 34
    dilution, 34
    immunoabsorption, 34

oxidation treatment, 11

peroxidase, 1, 13, 19
    development, 46, 48
peroxidase anti-peroxidase method, 20, 22,
        46
    advantages, 20
    disadvantage, 21
photomicrography, 44
poly-L-lysine, 12, 48
protease treatment, 10, 47
protein A, 27

quantification, 40

radioactive labels, 1, 13, 25
radioimmunoassay, 4, 7, 37
receptors, 41
region-specific antisera, 4, 6, 35

sensitivity
    enhancement of reaction, 12, 21, 47
    PAP method, 20
specificity problems, 33
streptavidin, 32

tissue preparation, 9
    adherence of sections to slides, 12, 48
    cryostat sections, 6, 8, 9, 47
    for electron microscopy, 10
    lipid breakdown, 9
    oxidation treatment, 11
    protease treatment, 10, 11, 47

unlabelled antibody-enzyme method, 20, 21

Plate 1. (top left) Cat pancreatic islet immunostained for insulin by the indirect immuno-fluorescence method using guinea pig anti-insulin as the first layer and fluoresceinconjugated rabbit anti-guinea pig IgG as the second layer. The periodic acid–Schiff counterstain which gives red background fluorescence was carried out before the immunostain. Tissue preparation: Tissue freeze-dried and fixed in p-benzoquinone vapour, then embedded in paraffin; 4 μm section. Photographed on Kodachrome 64.

Plate 2. (top right) Human pancreas. Double indirect immunoperoxidase stain by the Nakane method showing glucagon in brown and insulin in blue. The first antigen– antibody complex was eluted by acid, leaving insoluble brown DAB/peroxidase reaction product (glucagon cells) followed by an immunoperoxidase stain for insulin developed with 4-chloro-1-naphthol as the coupler, giving a blue reaction product. No counterstain. The section is mounted in an aqueous medium. Tissue preparation: Tissue freeze-dried and fixed in p-benzoquinone vapour, then embedded in paraffin; 4 μm section.

Plate 3. (centre left) Human pancreatic islet immunostained for glucagon by the peroxidase anti-peroxidase method. The peroxidase is developed in the amino ethylcarbazole medium giving a red reaction product (see A.4). Counterstained with haematoxylin. Tissue preparation: fixation in Bouin's solution followed by embedding in paraffin; 4 μm section.

Plate 4. (centre right) Human tonsil immunostained by the double immunoenzymatic method for kappa and lambda light immunoglobulin chains in plasma cells. The staining sequence was shown in Fig. 10. The mouse antibodies were kindly provided by Dr D. Y. Mason (Haematology Department, John Radcliffe Hospital, Oxford). Kappa chains stain brown (peroxidase–H_2O_2–DAB); lambda chains stain blue (alkaline phosphatase–naphthol AS-MX phosphate–Fast Blue BB). Note the mixed 'grey' colour of the extracellular immunoglobulin in the connective tissue. This indicates that the immunoglobulin is not synthesized in this tissue but has been absorbed indiscriminately from the environment and thus contains both kappa and lambda components. No counterstain; aqueous mountant. Tissue preparation: Tissue fixed in formol sublimate and embedded in paraffin; 4 μm section.

Plate 5. (bottom left) Dog pancreatic islet immunostained for glucagon by the peroxidase anti-peroxidase method. The peroxidase was developed in H_2O_2–DAB solution containing cobalt chloride. The end-product is intense blue-black. Tissue preparation: The tissue was freeze-dried and fixed in p-benzoquinone vapour, then embedded in paraffin; 4 μm section. Counterstained with neutral red.

Plate 6. (bottom right) Rat trachea (tangential section) immunostained for calcitonin gene-related peptide by the immunogold method with silver intensification. Note how well the fine nerve fibres stand out, even at this low magnification. Tissue preparation: fixation in Bouin's solution followed by embedding in paraffin; 4 μm section. Counterstained with haematoxylin and eosin.